Muscle Building

Quick and Easy Muscle Building and Fat Burning

(The Ultimate Guide to Strength Training - Essential Lifts for Muscle Building)

Joseph Gress

Published By **John Kembrey**

Joseph Gress

Muscle Building: Quick and Easy Muscle Building and Fat Burning (The Ultimate Guide to Strength Training - Essential Lifts for Muscle Building)

ISBN 978-0-9866928-7-1

No part of this guidebook shall be reproduced in any form without permission in writing from the publisher except in the case of brief quotations embodied in critical articles or reviews.

Legal & Disclaimer

Table Of Contents

Chapter 1: Understanding Muscle Anatomy 1

Chapter 2: Nutrition for Muscle Growth 15

Chapter 3: Strength Training Fundamentals 28

Chapter 4: Resistance Training Programs 40

Chapter 5: Muscle Recovery and Rest 55

Chapter 6: Supplements for Muscle Growth 67

Chapter 7: Tracking Progress 83

Chapter 8: Common Mistakes and How to Avoid Them 93

Chapter 9: Staying Motivated and Sustaining Gains 107

Chapter 10: Understanding Protein's Role 119

Chapter 11: Training Techniques 133

Chapter 12: Exercise Routine for Muscle Building 141

Chapter 13: The Importance of Cardiovascular Health in Men 145

Chapter 14: The Role of Rest and Recovery 155

Chapter 15: The Importance of Sleep for Men's Health.. 161

Chapter 16: Mental Health and Stress Management 173

Chapter 1: Understanding Muscle Anatomy

Muscles are essential components of the human frame, liable for movement, stability, and numerous physiological abilties. Understanding muscle anatomy and the manner muscle agencies art work is essential for all and sundry interested by health, sports activities sports, or human biology. Let's find out muscle anatomy and the mechanics of muscle contraction.

Muscle Anatomy:

Muscle Fibers: Muscles are composed of person muscle fibers, moreover known as muscle cells or myocytes. These fibers are the practical devices of muscle groups and are extended, cylindrical cells which can agreement to generate strain.

Fascicles: Muscle fibers are grouped together into bundles referred to as fascicles. Fascicles are wrapped in connective tissue layers that provide help and protection to the muscle.

Muscle Belly: The whole muscle, consisting of all its fascicles, makes up the muscle stomach. This is the seen, bulkier part of the muscle.

Tendons: At both ends of a muscle, the muscle fibers come collectively to shape a tendon. Tendons are dense connective tissues that join muscle groups to bones, permitting the muscle to transmit stress to the bone and produce motion.

Origin and Insertion: Muscles have primary factors of attachment: the start and the insertion. The starting location is the constant or heaps plenty less movable point wherein the muscle attaches to a bone, and the insertion is the movable attachment thing on each unique bone.

Agonist and Antagonist: In many muscle actions, there may be multiple muscle groups at paintings. The agonist (excessive mover) is the muscle chargeable for the popular motion, while the antagonist opposes that motion. For example, whilst you flex your biceps (agonist), your triceps (antagonist) lighten up.

Muscle Contraction:

Muscle contraction is a complex way concerning a sequence of physiological occasions. Here's an outline of the way muscle groups art work for the duration of contraction:

Neuromuscular Junction: The system begins while a nerve impulse, or motion capability, travels down a motor neuron to the neuromuscular junction, which is the element wherein the nerve meets the muscle fiber.

Release of Neurotransmitter: At the neuromuscular junction, the nerve releases a neurotransmitter known as acetylcholine (ACh). ACh binds to receptors on the muscle fiber's mobile membrane (sarcolemma).

Excitation: The binding of ACh to receptors triggers an electrical impulse that travels along the sarcolemma and into the muscle fiber via a community of tubules referred to as the T-tubules.

Calcium Release: The electric impulse in the T-tubules activates the discharge of calcium ions from a storage form known as the sarcoplasmic reticulum.

Cross-Bridge Formation: Calcium ions bind to a protein referred to as troponin, exposing binding web web sites on the skinny filaments of the muscle fiber. Myosin heads (thick filaments) then bind to those websites, forming skip-bridges.

Power Stroke: Energy from ATP is used to "cock" the myosin heads proper proper right into a excessive-electricity function. When calcium ions are gift, the myosin heads pivot, pulling the thin filaments within the path of the middle of the sarcomere, inflicting muscle contraction.

Sliding Filament Theory: Muscle contraction is frequently explained with the aid of using way of the sliding filament concept. It states that in contraction, the thin filaments (actin) slide over the thick filaments (myosin), shortening the sarcomere (the essential unit of muscle contraction) and ultimately the complete muscle fiber.

Relaxation: Muscle rest takes place whilst the worried stimulation ceases, and calcium ions are actively pumped once more into the sarcoplasmic reticulum. This causes the binding net internet web sites at the actin to be protected all another time, preventing further go-bridge formation.

Muscles paintings in a coordinated manner, contracting and relaxing to offer the extensive form of movements and forces wanted for severa sports. The frightened gadget performs a important feature in controlling those contractions, taking into account specific manipulate over muscle moves. Understanding muscle anatomy and body shape is fundamental to optimizing physical not unusual typical performance, preventing accidents, and selling regular health.

Types of muscle fibers and their role in energy and hypertrophy.

Muscles are composed of various sorts of muscle fibers, each with particular traits and roles in power and hypertrophy (muscle growth). There are by the usage of and huge 3 types of muscle fibers: Type I (sluggish-twitch), Type IIa (fast-twitch oxidative), and Type IIb (fast-twitch glycolytic). Understanding those fiber sorts is critical for tailoring your schooling to gain precise fitness dreams.

Type I (Slow-Twitch) Muscle Fibers:

Characteristics: Type I fibers are characterized with the beneficial resource of their gradual contraction speed, excessive resistance to fatigue, and reliance on cardio metabolism. They are rich in mitochondria (electricity-producing organelles) and myoglobin (oxygen-storing protein).

Role in Strength: Type I fibers are not properly-proper for maximal energy and strength sports activities sports because of the fact they generate decrease pressure outputs. However, they provide incredible staying power and are vital for sports like lengthy-distance strolling, cycling, and keeping posture.

Role in Hypertrophy: Type I fibers can undergo hypertrophy, but they reply higher to higher-repetition, decrease-load education. Endurance-oriented activities, which include strolling or swimming, can lead to 3 hypertrophy in Type I fibers because of prolonged muscle activation.

Type IIa (Fast-Twitch Oxidative) Muscle Fibers:

Characteristics: Type IIa fibers have a moderate contraction pace and resistance to fatigue. They use every cardio and anaerobic metabolism, making them bendy for numerous activities.

Role in Strength: Type IIa fibers play a super feature in power and power sports activities activities. They can produce higher strain outputs than Type I fibers and are crucial for sports like sprinting, leaping, and lifting weights.

Role in Hypertrophy: Type IIa fibers are aware of hypertrophy, and that they adapt nicely to resistance training. Moderate to heavy loads, at the aspect of mild repetitions (e.G., 6-12 reps in keeping with set), are powerful for stimulating hypertrophy in Type IIa fibers.

Type IIb (Fast-Twitch Glycolytic) Muscle Fibers:

Characteristics: Type IIb fibers agreement rapidly and are with out trouble fatigued. They depend carefully on anaerobic metabolism for strength production.

Role in Strength: Type IIb fibers are the most effective however also the quickest to fatigue. They are critical for short, excessive-depth efforts, collectively with lifting heavy weights explosively or appearing brief sprints.

Role in Hypertrophy: Type IIb fibers can hypertrophy appreciably in reaction to resistance training, in particular with heavy loads and occasional repetitions (e.G., 1-6 reps in step with set). This form of schooling is robust for maximizing muscle length and energy.

To optimize power and hypertrophy earnings, it's far important to bear in mind your training desires and encompass some of training techniques:

Strength Focus: To target Type IIa and Type IIb fibers for electricity profits, encompass heavy resistance training with low to slight repetitions (1-6 reps for maximum power, 6-12 reps for electricity-staying power).

Hypertrophy Focus: For muscle hypertrophy, emphasize mild to heavy hundreds with slight to higher repetitions (6-12 reps). Vary your bodily games and training quantity to aim brilliant muscle fiber sorts.

Endurance Focus: If your purpose is endurance, include longer-duration, lower-intensity sports activities like taking walks, cycling, or swimming, that allows you to on the entire engage Type I fibers.

In precis, information the sorts of muscle fibers and their roles in electricity and hypertrophy is critical for designing an effective training utility. By tailoring your workout sporting events to intention precise fiber types, you may gain your fitness dreams greater correctly and efficiently.

Importance of right muscle activation in the course of training.

Proper muscle activation in the course of education is of paramount importance for reaching health goals, preventing accidents, and maximizing the effectiveness of your exercise workouts. Here are numerous key reasons why proper muscle activation is vital:

Efficient Workouts: Activating the aim muscle businesses guarantees that they will be doing the bulk of the art work in some unspecified time in the destiny of an exercising. This overall performance approach which you get the most out of your workout in phrases of muscle improvement and energy profits.

Targeted Muscle Growth: To stimulate muscle boom (hypertrophy) in a specific muscle employer, it's miles crucial to set off the ones muscle groups absolutely. Proper activation guarantees which you are placing the essential strain at the muscle fibers to stimulate increase.

Injury Prevention: Activating the correct muscle businesses permits stabilize and protect joints. When the encompassing muscle businesses art work as they want to, they lessen the strain on ligaments and tendons, reducing the threat of injuries.

Improved Performance: Proper muscle activation can enhance your athletic performance. It lets in you to generate extra pressure and electricity, whether or not or no longer you are lifting weights, jogging, jumping, or collaborating in sports sports.

Balanced Muscle Development: Ensuring that each one muscle agencies are activated well promotes balanced muscle development. Muscle imbalances can reason postural troubles and growth the danger of harm.

Enhanced Mind-Muscle Connection: Focusing on muscle activation cultivates a sturdy thoughts-muscle connection. This heightened attention allows you to revel in and control your muscles higher, this is in particular beneficial in sports activities that require precision and control.

Reduced Compensation Patterns: When muscle mass are not activated efficaciously, one of a kind muscle tissues regularly compensate to perform the movement. Over time, those reimbursement patterns can cause overuse injuries and save you development in energy and information improvement.

Functional Fitness: Proper muscle activation is important for useful health. It allows you perform every day duties with greater ease and general performance, which includes lifting, bending, and achieving.

Improved Muscle Endurance: By activating muscle organizations effectively, you may enhance their staying strength. Muscles which might be accustomed to working effectively are an entire lot less in all likelihood to fatigue short.

Customized Training: Proper activation lets in you to tailor your training to specific dreams. You can emphasize the activation of great muscle groups to work on weaknesses or address person health objectives.

To ensure proper muscle activation sooner or later of training:

Warm-Up: Always begin your exercising with a right warmness-up that includes dynamic stretching and mobility bodily sports activities. This prepares your muscle businesses for extra excessive activation.

Focus on Form: Pay close to hobby on your exercise form and approach. Proper shape helps ensure that the right muscle corporations are activated and decreases the chance of damage.

Mind-Muscle Connection: Concentrate on the muscle tissue you are targeted on for the duration of every exercising. Visualize the muscle contracting and actively interact it in the course of the movement.

Chapter 2: Nutrition for Muscle Growth

Nutrition performs a essential role in muscle constructing, and it's miles regularly stated that "abs are made in the kitchen." Proper nutrients gives the critical building blocks and strength required for muscle growth and healing. Here's an in depth explanation of the characteristic of vitamins in muscle building:

Protein Intake: Protein is the cornerstone of muscle constructing. When you interact in resistance schooling or specific kinds of workout, you create microscopic tears to your muscle fibers. Consuming an true sufficient amount of protein gives the amino acids vital for repairing and building those muscle fibers, ensuing in muscle increase. The recommended protein intake varies but is usually spherical zero.8 to at least one.2 grams of protein steady with pound of frame weight in line with day for those engaged in energy education.

Caloric Surplus: To collect muscle, you want to devour more energy than your frame burns in a day, creating a caloric surplus. This surplus presents the strength desired for muscle restore and increase. However, it is vital to strike the proper stability, as excessive calorie consumption can reason fat benefit.

Carbohydrates: Carbohydrates are your body's number one supply of strength. They provide the gasoline required for intense exercises and pinnacle off glycogen shops in muscle corporations after workout. Carbohydrates furthermore spare protein from being used as an energy supply, preserving it for muscle growth and repair.

Healthy Fats: Dietary fats are important for everyday health and hormone production. Healthy fats, inclusive of these determined in avocados, nuts, and fatty fish, can guide muscle-constructing efforts and optimize hormone balance, this is essential for muscle boom.

Micronutrients: Vitamins and minerals, regularly known as micronutrients, play vital roles in muscle building. For example, diet D allows muscle function and bone health, even as minerals like magnesium and zinc are involved in protein synthesis and muscle contractions. A nicely-balanced weight loss plan rich in end result, vegetables, and whole grains guarantees you obtain an array of micronutrients.

Timing of Nutrient Intake:

Pre-Workout: Consuming a balanced meal with carbohydrates and protein in advance than a exercise gives power and amino acids for muscle help.

Post-Workout: After exercising, your muscle mass are primed for nutrient uptake. Consuming a mixture of carbohydrates and protein within the first couple of hours placed up-exercise can enhance muscle healing and boom.

Throughout the Day: Distribute your protein consumption calmly in the course of the day to maintain a consistent deliver of amino acids for muscle restore and boom.

Hydration: Staying well-hydrated is critical for muscle characteristic and regular fitness. Dehydration can result in muscle cramps and decrease workout ordinary universal performance. Water is also required for numerous metabolic techniques, such as protein synthesis.

Supplementation: While whole food ought to be your number one supply of vitamins, a few human beings also can advantage from unique nutritional dietary supplements like protein powder, creatine, or branched-chain amino acids (BCAAs) to assist muscle constructing. Always speak over with a healthcare expert earlier than consisting of nutritional nutritional supplements for your habitual.

Rest and Recovery: Adequate sleep and relaxation are frequently ignored but critical aspects of muscle constructing. During deep sleep, the frame releases boom hormone, which performs a considerable feature in muscle restore and increase.

In summary, vitamins is a cornerstone of muscle constructing. To maximize your muscle-building efforts, attention on eating an ok quantity of protein, keeping a caloric surplus, and fueling your frame with a balanced healthy dietweight-reduction plan wealthy in carbohydrates, healthy fats, and micronutrients. Additionally, taking note of nutrient timing and staying well hydrated are key additives of a a success muscle-building vitamins plan.

Macronutrients and their importance.

Macronutrients are the 3 essential instructions of vitamins that offer strength and are vital for the right functioning of the human frame. These macronutrients are carbohydrates, proteins, and fats. Each macronutrient has a completely unique characteristic and importance in keeping popular health and nicely-being:

Carbohydrates: Significance: Carbohydrates are the frame's number one supply of strength. They provide the glucose had to fuel numerous physiological techniques, which incorporates thoughts feature, muscle contractions, and each day sports sports.

Role: Carbohydrates are broken down into glucose, which may be used without delay for energy or stored inside the muscle groups and liver as glycogen for future use. In addition to imparting strength, carbohydrates additionally play a function in keeping right digestive feature and helping healthy metabolism.

Types: Carbohydrates are available in two critical paperwork: complex and simple. Complex carbohydrates, decided in food like entire grains, greens, and legumes, offer sustained electricity due to their slower digestion. Simple carbohydrates, discovered in sugars and processed components, offer quick bursts of energy.

Recommended Intake: The advocated every day consumption of carbohydrates varies but commonly constitutes approximately forty five-sixty 5% of regularly occurring every day power.

Proteins:

Significance: Proteins are essential for the increase, restore, and maintenance of tissues in the body. They play a large function in building and repairing muscle tissue, organs, enzymes, hormones, and antibodies.

Role: Proteins are made from amino acids, which can be the constructing blocks of the body. Different mixtures of amino acids create diverse proteins with precise competencies. Essential amino acids need to be obtained from the weight loss program because of the fact the frame can not synthesize them.

Sources: Protein-rich substances encompass meat, poultry, fish, dairy merchandise, eggs, legumes, nuts, and seeds.

Recommended Intake: The endorsed every day consumption of protein varies primarily based on factors which include age, interest degree, and essential health. For maximum adults, protein ought to make up approximately 10-35% of standard each day energy.

Fats:

Significance: Fats serve numerous vital skills within the frame. They offer a targeted supply of electricity, useful resource mobile increase, protect organs, useful aid in the absorption of fat-soluble nutrients (A, D, E, and K), and play a function in hormone manufacturing.

Role: Fats are crafted from fatty acids, which can be categorised as saturated, unsaturated (monounsaturated and polyunsaturated), and trans fat. Healthy fats, like monounsaturated and polyunsaturated fats determined in avocados, olive oil, and fatty fish, help coronary heart fitness, even as saturated and trans fat, found in lots of processed ingredients, may have bad fitness effects at the identical time as ate up in greater.

Sources: Healthy fats assets embody nuts, seeds, fatty fish (e.G., salmon and mackerel), avocados, and olive oil.

Recommended Intake: Dietary guidelines typically suggest that fats make up about 20-35% of wellknown every day energy, with a focus on ingesting basically unsaturated fats.

Balancing the consumption of those macronutrients is critical for keeping a wholesome food regimen and selling ordinary properly-being. Individual nutritional desires can range based totally mostly on elements like age, hobby degree, and health desires, so it's useful to talk over with a registered dietitian or healthcare issuer to create a customised nutritional plan that meets your precise requirements.

Creating a muscle-building diet plan and facts calorie desires.

Creating a muscle-building diet plan includes expertise your calorie goals, macronutrient ratios, and meal timing to assist muscle boom efficaciously. Here's a step-through-step guide:

1. Calculate Your Daily Calorie Needs:

Determine your Total Daily Energy Expenditure (TDEE), which incorporates your Basal Metabolic Rate (BMR) and hobby diploma. Your BMR is the sort of energy your body goals at rest. You can use a web calculator to estimate your TDEE. Once you have got your TDEE, add more energy to create a caloric surplus, commonly within the variety of 250-500 energy in step with day. This surplus provides the strength wished for muscle boom.

2. Set Your Protein Intake:

Protein is crucial for muscle repair and boom. Aim for round 1.Zero to as a minimum one.2 grams of protein regular with pound of body weight every day. Divide your protein intake calmly at some point of your food to make certain a steady deliver of amino acids.

three. Determine Your Fat Intake:

Include healthy fat to your diet as they help installed health and hormone production. A favored guiding precept is to allocate about 20-35% of your each day strength to fats. Focus on unsaturated fat, which incorporates those decided in avocados, nuts, and olive oil.

4. Allocate Carbohydrates:

The remaining strength will come from carbohydrates. Carbs are crucial for strength inside the route of exercising workouts and for replenishing glycogen stores in muscle tissue. The particular carb intake varies based totally on individual alternatives and hobby levels. A not unusual variety is 45-65% of ordinary every day energy.

five. Plan Your Meals:

Pre-Workout: Consume a balanced meal 1-2 hours earlier than your workout. Include carbs for energy and protein to assist muscle feature. A sample pre-exercise meal might be grilled fowl breast with brown rice and steamed greens.

Post-Workout: After exercise, have a meal or snack containing every protein and carbohydrates to useful useful resource recuperation and muscle restore. A protein shake with a banana is a short and effective opportunity.

Other Meals: Include lean belongings of protein (e.G., hen, fish, tofu), complicated carbohydrates (e.G., whole grains, sweet potatoes), and wholesome fats (e.G., avocado, nuts) to your extraordinary food and snacks. Try to devour every three-four hours to offer a steady supply of nutrients for muscle increase.

6. Stay Hydrated:

Adequate hydration is essential for regular fitness and muscle characteristic. Aim to drink hundreds of water sooner or later of the day, and maintain in thoughts a sports activities sports drink with electrolytes at some point of extreme exercise workouts.

7. Monitor Your Progress:

Regularly song your development through assessing your muscle benefit and body composition. Adjust your calorie consumption and macronutrient ratios primarily based completely to your outcomes. If you aren't making the desired development, keep in mind developing your caloric surplus or adjusting your macronutrient ratios.

8. Be Patient and Consistent:

Building muscle takes time, so be affected person and live normal in conjunction with your eating regimen and training. Make changes as needed, and consider that proper sleep and recovery are also essential components of muscle boom.

It's vital to be aware that individual calorie wishes and macronutrient ratios can also moreover variety primarily based on elements like metabolism, age, gender, and interest diploma. Consulting with a registered dietitian or nutritionist allow you to create a customized muscle-constructing diet regime tailored for your precise goals and dreams.

Chapter 3: Strength Training Fundamentals

Strength education is a foundational element of fitness that specializes in constructing and enhancing muscular power, patience, and electricity. Understanding the requirements of electricity training is vital for designing effective exercise applications and accomplishing your health dreams. Here's an creation to the ones key thoughts:

Progressive Overload: This precept workplace paintings the inspiration of energy schooling. It involves gradually growing the resistance or intensity of your exercising workouts over time. By continually tough your muscle mass with gradually heavier weights or more resistance, you stimulate muscle increase and strength income.

Specificity: The precept of specificity emphasizes that the schooling outcomes are particular to the form of workout and muscle organizations labored. To enhance in a selected area (e.G., higher frame power or staying power), you must perform sports sports centered on those precise muscle groups or moves.

Volume: Volume refers back to the complete quantity of hard work completed in a training consultation and is typically calculated via multiplying gadgets, reps, and weight lifted. Manipulating extent let you gain diverse training results, alongside side hypertrophy (muscle growth) with higher quantity or electricity profits with lower quantity and heavier weights.

Intensity: Intensity is the amount of resistance or weight lifted relative in your one-repetition maximum (1RM), it absolutely is the maximum weight you may beautify for a single repetition. Adjusting the intensity stage could have an impact on whether or not or no longer your schooling specializes in power, endurance, or hypertrophy.

Rest and Recovery: Adequate rest and recuperation are essential for muscle repair and increase. Strength schooling creates microtears in muscle fibers, and healing periods permit the ones fibers to heal and come to be more potent. Proper sleep, vitamins, and lively healing techniques are vital for optimizing healing.

Variation: Introducing variety into your electricity training everyday prevents plateaus and maintains workout physical activities attractive. Changing physical activities, rep schemes, and schooling modalities (e.G., unfastened weights, machines, body weight physical sports) can stimulate muscle boom and enhance standard energy.

Form and Technique: Maintaining right form and approach is vital to prevent injuries and optimize the effectiveness of your physical games. Focus on acting carrying activities with accurate posture, alignment, and variety of motion.

Frequency: The frequency of your strength training intervals can variety based totally in your desires and fitness diploma. Beginners can also start with 2-3 schooling in step with week, at the same time as more superior people may moreover teach 4-6 times in step with week. Consistency is fundamental for conducting outcomes.

Periodization: Periodization is a scientific approach to organizing your education into wonderful levels or cycles. Each section has precise dreams and schooling variables, which consist of volume and intensity, that change over time to keep away from version plateaus.

Recovery and Deload Weeks: Incorporating recuperation and deload weeks into your training plan permits your frame to recover absolutely, lowering the threat of overtraining and burnout. During the ones weeks, you reduce the schooling quantity and depth to provide your muscles a spoil.

Nutrition: Proper nutrients is vital for fueling your workout routines and helping muscle increase and recovery. Consume a balanced food plan with an proper enough intake of protein, carbohydrates, and wholesome fat to meet your power and nutrient goals.

Understanding and making use of these strength training thoughts will help you create powerful workout applications, set practicable goals, and make normal improvement in building power, muscle groups, and normal health. Whether you're a beginner or an professional lifter, the ones standards form the concept for secure and successful strength education.

Importance of right form and method.

Proper shape and approach are essential factors of any exercising or bodily hobby. Whether you are lifting weights, acting frame weight sporting sports, or accomplishing sports activities, preserving accurate form and approach is of most importance. Here's why right shape and approach are essential:

Injury Prevention: Proper shape reduces the danger of accidents extensively. When you operate incorrect method, you may place immoderate stress on joints, ligaments, tendons, and muscle mass, fundamental to sprains, lines, and further severe accidents. For instance, lifting weights with a rounded decrease returned can stress your spine, at the equal time as wrong walking form can cause knee or hip injuries.

Efficiency: Correct form and approach will let you perform physical video games and actions greater successfully. When you float efficiently, you operate a good deal less strength and decrease useless stress in your frame. This performance is specially vital in sports sports and staying power sports activities wherein preserving power can enhance universal overall performance.

Muscle Engagement: Proper form ensures that the focused muscle groups are engaged efficiently in some unspecified time in the future of an exercise. This results in better muscle recruitment and development. Incorrect shape can shift the emphasis to the wrong muscle businesses or bring about muscle imbalances.

Strength and Progression: Proper approach is critical for building energy and making development to your bodily activities. When you operate proper form, you can deliver heavier weights or perform greater repetitions, number one to more muscle stimulation and growth.

Functional Movement: Many physical sports and moves in strength education and sports activities activities mimic useful sports in each day existence. Proper shape inside the route of those carrying occasions allows decorate your ordinary sensible fitness, making it much less difficult to carry out every day duties and decrease the threat of damage in ordinary sports activities.

Skill Development: In sports sports and bodily sports activities sports, right method is critical for skills development and mastery. Skillful execution allows athletes to carry out at their exceptional and compete successfully.

Long-Term Health: Consistently the usage of proper shape and technique for your workout exercises and sports activities can make a contribution to prolonged-time period joint health and decrease the hazard of chronic problems like arthritis, joint degeneration, and decrease decrease back ache.

Mental Focus: Focusing on proper form and approach enhances your thoughts-muscle connection. This intellectual engagement let you stay stimulated, hold attention, and make exercise routines extra powerful.

Injury Rehabilitation: If you are recuperating from an damage, maintaining proper shape within the path of rehabilitation bodily sports is essential for a solid and a success healing. It ensures that you intention the injured region correctly at the same time as minimizing the danger of re-harm.

Confidence and Self-Efficacy: Achieving proper shape and method gives you a revel in of accomplishment and self assurance on your skills. This self belief can translate into better normal overall performance and a extra superb attitude in the direction of fitness and physical interest.

To ensure proper form and approach:

Start with lighter weights or resistance and little by little development as you grow to be greater gifted.

Seek steerage from a certified fitness expert or teach to study right technique for unique sporting sports or sports.

Use mirrors or video recordings to assess and refine your shape.

Listen on your body and be privy to any discomfort or pain, which can be a sign of wrong technique.

Ultimately, proper form and approach are vital for maximizing the blessings of exercising, minimizing the danger of damage, and promoting prolonged-time period fitness and health. Whether you are a novice or an skilled athlete, usually prioritize form and technique for your schooling normal.

Different kinds of resistance schooling (unfastened weights, machines, body weight).

Resistance education, additionally called energy schooling or weight training, includes the use of severa forms of resistance to artwork towards the pressure of gravity, most important to muscle improvement and strength earnings. There are numerous varieties of resistance schooling, each with its private advantages and dispositions. Here are the 3 number one types:

Free Weights:

Definition: Free weights encompass dumbbells, barbells, and kettlebells. These are unattached weights that allow for a giant form of movement.

Advantages:

Functional Strength: Free weights require more stabilization and engagement of supporting muscle agencies, primary to beneficial power earnings.

Versatility: They offer a huge shape of bodily video games, allowing you to goal precise muscle agencies or carry out compound actions.

Balance and Coordination: Using loose weights demanding situations balance and coordination, promoting progressed motor skills.

Examples: Dumbbell bench press, barbell squat, kettlebell swing, bicep curls with dumbbells.

Machines:

Definition: Resistance machines have a predefined form of motion and a tough and rapid route for the weights. They are generally found in gyms and health facilities.

Advantages:

Safety: Machines are frequently considered extra steady for beginners due to the truth they provide assist and manipulate over the burden.

Isolation: They allow for focused muscle isolation, making them useful for rehabilitation and addressing muscle imbalances.

Ease of Use: Machines are individual-exceptional and require lots less knowledge and balance in evaluation to loose weights.

Examples: Leg press machine, chest press device, lat pulldown device.

Chapter 4: Resistance Training Programs

Resistance education packages are primarily based exercising plans that target building energy, muscle businesses, and staying power. These programs can be tailor-made to character dreams and alternatives. Here's a top level view of various resistance education application kinds:

Full-Body Workout:

Overview: Full-body workout physical activities purpose all most important muscle businesses in a single session. They are commonly carried out 2-3 instances in keeping with week.

Advantages:

Time-Efficient: Fewer workout workouts consistent with week, making it suitable for busy schedules.

Balanced Muscle Development: Ensures that every one muscle agencies collect hobby.

Great for Beginners: A truthful technique for the ones new to energy education.

Example Exercises: Squats, deadlifts, bench presses, pull-ups, and lunges.

Split Routines:

Overview: Split physical activities divide muscle agencies into excellent exercising days. Common splits include:

Upper/Lower Split: Alternates among upper body and reduce frame workouts.

Push/Pull Split: Separates pushing (chest, shoulders, triceps) and pulling (lower returned, biceps) bodily video video games.

Muscle Group Split: Dedicates every exercise to a particular muscle organisation (e.G., chest, lower once more, legs, arms, shoulders).

Advantages:

Allows for extra quantity consistent with muscle group, doubtlessly primary to more muscle improvement.

Ideal for advanced lifters seeking to specialise in high satisfactory areas.

Permits healing of particular muscle agencies amongst physical games.

Example Exercises: Upper body: bench press, bicep curls, tricep dips. Lower body: squats, lunges, calf will increase.

Strength and Power Programs:

Overview: These applications attention on growing maximal power and electricity. They frequently contain lower rep degrees (1-6 reps in keeping with set) and heavy weights.

Advantages:

Ideal for athletes and powerlifters trying to find to increase their one-rep max (1RM).

Builds explosive power and velocity.

Typically shorter carrying activities because of low rep tiers.

Example Exercises: Powerlifting movements (squat, bench press, deadlift), Olympic lifts (grab, clean and jerk), plyometrics (situation jumps, medicinal drug ball throws).

Hypertrophy Programs:

Overview: Hypertrophy applications awareness on muscle growth. They frequently contain mild rep tiers (6-12 reps consistent with set) and a mild to immoderate quantity of wearing sports activities.

Advantages:

Maximizes muscle length and definition.

Suitable for bodybuilders and those interested in aesthetics.

Typically includes greater isolation sports sports to aim particular muscle tissue.

Example Exercises: Dumbbell curls, leg press, lateral will increase, cable flyes, machine bodily video games.

Endurance Programs:

Overview: These packages emphasize muscular persistence, frequently associated with immoderate rep degrees (12+ reps in keeping with set) and shorter relaxation intervals amongst gadgets.

Advantages:

Enhances the functionality to maintain muscular strive over the years.

Useful for athletes in sports requiring prolonged bodily exertion (e.G., biking, swimming).

Can assist beautify cardiovascular health at the same time as mixed with aerobic workout.

Example Exercises: Bodyweight physical activities (push-ups, planks, body weight squats), circuit education, resistance band carrying activities.

Functional Training:

Overview: Functional education focuses on actions that mimic actual-existence activities. It emphasizes balance, stability, and center electricity.

Advantages:

Improves regular useful health and athleticism.

Reduces the risk of damage at some stage in every day sports activities.

Ideal for those looking to improve their physical general performance specially sports activities sports or sports.

Example Exercises: Medicine ball throws, TRX suspension schooling, balance ball carrying activities, agility ladder drills.

The preference of a resistance education application ought to align collectively together with your desires, revel in stage, and personal alternatives. Many individuals include masses of those software program program kinds at a few level inside the twelve months to sell properly-rounded fitness and prevent plateaus in their improvement. Additionally, it is critical to conform and adjust your application as you improvement to maintain challenging your frame and wearing out your fitness goals.

How to design a custom designed exercise utility.

Designing a personalized workout utility consists of tailoring your exercising everyday to your unique desires, health stage, and alternatives. Here's a step-by means of manner of-step guide to help you create an powerful and individualized exercising plan:

1. Set Clear Goals:

Define your health dreams. Are you trying to construct muscle, shed pounds, enhance staying energy, growth strength, or beautify standard fitness? Having clean desires will guide your software format.

2. Assess Your Current Fitness Level:

Evaluate your modern-day-day health diploma and bear in mind any boundaries or medical conditions. Assess your electricity, patience, flexibility, and cardiovascular fitness. This evaluation will assist you select suitable sporting sports and progressions.

three. Choose Your Workout Frequency:

Determine what number of days in line with week you may determine to running out. For beginners, 2-three days in step with week is a good start line. More skilled people can also teach 4-6 days in keeping with week. Make certain to encompass rest days for recovery.

4. Select the Type of Training:

Depending in your dreams, choose the form of schooling that aligns with them. Common options encompass:

Strength Training: For building muscle and power.

Cardiovascular Training: For improving staying power and cardiovascular fitness.

Flexibility and Mobility Training: To enhance flexibility and joint kind of motion.

Functional Training: To enhance popular beneficial fitness and athleticism.

High-Intensity Interval Training (HIIT): For a aggregate of energy and cardio benefits.

five. Choose Exercises:

Select sports activities that focus on the muscle corporations or fitness additives applicable to your desires. Include compound carrying sports (multi-joint movements) and isolation bodily video games (unmarried-joint moves) as wanted. Ensure variety to save you boredom and overuse accidents.

6. Determine Sets and Repetitions:

Set the huge form of gadgets and repetitions (reps) for every exercising. The significant guiding principle is:

Strength and hypertrophy: three-five units of 6-12 reps

Endurance: 2-4 units of 12-20+ reps

Strength and strength: 3-6 gadgets of one-6 reps

7. Plan Rest Intervals:

Determine how lengthy you may relaxation amongst gadgets and sporting events. Shorter relaxation periods (30 seconds to one minute) emphasize persistence, at the equal time as longer rests (2-3 minutes) are appropriate for electricity and hypertrophy schooling.

eight. Establish Progression:

Incorporate a development plan to typically project your frame. This can also comprise growing weight, reps, devices, or intensity as you switch out to be more skilled.

9. Create a Workout Schedule:

Outline your weekly exercising time table, consisting of the instances you will exercising, the form of exercise workouts you can do (e.G., power on Monday, cardio on Wednesday), and an appropriate sports activities for every workout.

10. Warm-Up and Cool-Down:

Include warm-up wearing activities to put together your frame for the exercising and funky-down stretches to enhance flexibility and reduce muscle discomfort publish-workout.

eleven. Track Your Progress:

Keep a workout magazine or use fitness apps to file your exercises, which incorporates weights lifted, reps, devices, and any notes approximately the manner you felt at a few diploma within the consultation. Tracking development allows you're making adjustments and stay stimulated.

12. Listen to Your Body:

Pay interest to how your frame responds to this machine. If you enjoy pain, fatigue, or ache, alter your exercise physical activities therefore and bear in mind consulting a health expert or healthcare agency.

thirteen. Nutrition and Recovery:

Support your exercising software with a balanced food regimen that meets your power and nutrient desires. Prioritize sleep and recovery strategies, which embody appropriate sufficient relaxation, hydration, and stretching.

14. Seek Professional Guidance:

Consider operating with an authorized non-public teacher or health professional, especially if you're new to workout or have unique dreams or boundaries. They can provide personalised steering, shape tests, and expert advice.

Remember that designing a customized exercising software program is an ongoing approach. As you development and adapt, be open to growing changes in your plan to make sure it maintains to align together collectively together with your evolving fitness desires and desires.

Periodization and improvement for non-forestall earnings.

Periodization and development are critical necessities in designing a exercise utility that enables non-prevent earnings in strength, muscle size, endurance, and everyday fitness. They involve systematically numerous and developing the training variables over time to keep away from plateaus and optimize trendy basic overall performance. Here's how periodization and improvement paintings collectively to obtain non-prevent profits:

1. Periodization:

Periodization is a set up approach to organizing your schooling into extremely good stages or cycles. Each phase has specific dreams and training variables that trade over the years. The number one motive of periodization is to prevent model plateaus, lessen the hazard of overtraining, and sell prolonged-term development.

Components of Periodization:

Macrocycles: These are the longest education cycles, often spanning severa months to a 365 days. They are divided into smaller ranges.

Mesocycles: These intermediate cycles generally final some weeks to three months and characteristic precise training focuses, which includes strength, hypertrophy, or endurance.

Microcycles: Microcycles are the shortest training cycles, commonly lasting in keeping with week. They contain the each day or weekly exercising sports, together with sets, reps, and physical activities.

Types of Periodization:

Linear Periodization: In this model, training variables like depth (weight), amount (gadgets and reps), and rest durations gradually alternate in a linear fashion. For instance, you could start with higher reps and reduce weights and step by step shift to lower reps and heavier weights.

Chapter 5: Muscle Recovery and Rest

Rest and recuperation are necessary additives of any muscle-building application. While immoderate workout workouts are essential for stimulating muscle growth, it's far at some point of the intervals of relaxation and recuperation that your frame definitely maintenance and strengthens the muscle fibers, taking into consideration non-stop development. Here's why relaxation and recuperation are so crucial in muscle building:

Muscle Repair and Growth: When you engage in resistance education or energy carrying sports, you create micro-tears for your muscle fibers. These microscopic injuries are essential for muscle growth. During the relaxation and recuperation segment, your frame maintenance those tears thru fusing muscle fibers collectively, making them thicker and stronger. This manner is what in the long run effects in muscle growth and progressed strength.

Hormone Production: Rest and sleep are important for the release of essential hormones worried in muscle building. One of the maximum important hormones is growth hormone (GH), this is launched for the duration of deep sleep. GH performs a large function in tissue restore, muscle increase, and fashionable healing.

Energy Restoration: Intense physical video games expend your frame's power shops, specifically glycogen (stored carbohydrates) to your muscle tissue. Proper rest and recovery allow your body to pinnacle off the ones power stores, ensuring you've got were given the gas wanted in your subsequent workout.

Reduction of Muscle Soreness: Rest permits for the treatment of muscle soreness and contamination, that would rise up after immoderate wearing activities. During this time, your frame renovation damaged tissues and eliminates waste products, along with lactic acid, from the muscle businesses.

Injury Prevention: Overtraining or no longer allowing top enough rest can bring about overuse accidents, fatigue, and a better threat of accidents because of decreased coordination and interest. Rest allows prevent the ones problems and decreases the danger of injuries.

Central Nervous System Recovery: Intense exercise routines additionally area strain for your vital anxious machine (CNS). Rest and healing are critical on your CNS to move again to an maximum green kingdom, making sure that you may perform at your best in subsequent exercise workouts.

Mental Well-Being: Physical and highbrow fatigue can accumulate with out enough rest. Adequate recuperation time allows lessen intellectual fatigue, enhance temper, and beautify motivation, which is probably crucial for prolonged-time period consistency on your education utility.

Tips for Effective Rest and Recovery in Muscle Building:

Sleep: Aim for 7-9 hours of great sleep in keeping with night time time time, as deep sleep is while most of the body's repair and boom methods get up.

Nutrition: Consume a well-balanced weight-reduction plan with an emphasis on protein and carbohydrates to assist muscle restoration and pinnacle off strength shops.

Active Recovery: Light, low-intensity sports like strolling, swimming, or yoga on relaxation days can promote blood go along with the waft and decrease muscle pain.

Hydration: Stay thoroughly hydrated to manual all physiological approaches, which incorporates muscle restore.

Stretching and Mobility Work: Incorporate stretching and mobility bodily video games to improve flexibility and save you muscle imbalances.

Rest Days: Schedule everyday rest days into your training application to permit your muscle groups and nervous tool to without a doubt get higher.

Listen to Your Body: Pay attention to signs and symptoms of overtraining, collectively with continual fatigue, continual ache, and decreased traditional performance. If you word the ones signs and symptoms, maintain in thoughts adjusting your schooling quantity or intensity and permitting greater time for restoration.

In precis, relaxation and healing are vital for muscle building and everyday fitness. They promote muscle restore, hormone production, and energy restoration even as decreasing the chance of damage and enhancing highbrow nicely-being. A well-balanced technique to education that includes ok relaxation and recovery is pinnacle to attaining prolonged-term achievement on your muscle-building journey.

Strategies for optimizing healing, together with sleep and nutrients.

Optimizing restoration is essential for everyday fitness, muscle growth, and athletic performance. Two key components of healing are sleep and nutrients. Here are techniques to optimize each:

1. Sleep:

Quality sleep is essential for recuperation and average well-being. It's for the duration of sleep that your frame preservation tissues, releases boom hormone, and consolidates reminiscences. Here's the manner to optimize your sleep for higher recuperation:

Consistent Sleep Schedule: Go to mattress and awaken on the same time every day, even on weekends. This lets in alter your frame's internal clock.

Create a Relaxing Bedtime Routine: Wind down in advance than mattress with the resource of the usage of sporting out calming sports activities together with analyzing, stretching, or deep respiratory bodily video games.

Dark and Cool Sleep Environment: Keep your mattress room dark, quiet, and at a fab, cushty temperature. Consider the use of blackout curtains and earplugs if important.

Limit Screen Time: Reduce publicity to presentations (telephones, pills, computer structures, TVs) as a minimum an hour earlier than bedtime. The blue mild emitted by using manner of video show devices can intervene with the producing of melatonin, a hormone that regulates sleep.

Avoid Stimulants: Avoid caffeine and nicotine inside the hours principal as a great deal as bedtime, as they are able to disrupt sleep styles.

Limit Fluid Intake Before Bed: Minimize your consumption of fluids in the night time time to reduce the chance of waking up for bathroom journeys at a few level in the night time time.

Regular Exercise: Engage in regular bodily interest, however try to complete your exercise severa hours earlier than bedtime. Exercise can promote higher sleep, however exercising too close to bedtime can also have the other effect.

Limit Alcohol: While alcohol must make you revel in sleepy to start with, it may disrupt sleep patterns and motive poorer-excellent rest.

Manage Stress: Practice rest techniques consisting of meditation or contemporary muscle relaxation to reduce pressure and anxiety that can intervene with sleep.

Consult a Healthcare Professional: If you have got have been given persistent sleep problems, keep in mind searching out recommendation from a healthcare professional or sleep expert.

2. Nutrition:

Proper nutrients plays a massive feature in healing by means of manner of manner of offering the vital nutrients for muscle restore and energy replenishment. Here are nutrients techniques to optimize recuperation:

Balanced Diet: Consume a well-balanced eating regimen that includes a number of meals, which include lean protein sources, complex carbohydrates, healthful fats, and masses of prevent cease result and veggies.

Protein Intake: Protein is essential for muscle restore and increase. Ensure you have become an ok amount of protein from sources like lean meats, hen, fish, dairy, eggs, legumes, and plant-based totally resources like tofu and tempeh.

Carbohydrates: Carbohydrates are vital for replenishing glycogen shops in muscle groups. Include complex carbohydrates like whole grains, candy potatoes, and quinoa in your post-exercise food.

Hydration: Stay properly hydrated with the aid of eating hundreds of water throughout the day. Proper hydration enables all physiological procedures, which encompass muscle restoration.

Post-Workout Nutrition: After exercising, consume a balanced meal or snack that includes every protein and carbohydrates to assist healing. This may be a protein shake with a banana or a turkey sandwich on whole-grain bread.

Omega-3 Fatty Acids: Include belongings of omega-three fatty acids, collectively with fatty fish (salmon, mackerel), flaxseeds, chia seeds, and walnuts, as they've got anti-inflammatory residences that would useful resource in restoration.

Antioxidant-Rich Foods: Consume meals excessive in antioxidants, collectively with berries, dark leafy veggies, and colourful greens, to help lessen workout-brought on oxidative stress.

Meal Timing: Spread your meals inside the path of the day to offer a consistent deliver of nutrients for recuperation. Eating a aggregate of protein and carbohydrates within 1-2 hours after exercise is particularly critical.

Supplements: Consider consulting with a healthcare expert or registered dietitian to decide if dietary dietary supplements like creatine, branched-chain amino acids (BCAAs), or protein powders are appropriate on your recovery goals.

By prioritizing each sleep and nutrients, you can optimize your restoration and assist your fitness desires. These techniques aren't top notch useful for athletes but additionally for everybody seeking to guide a healthful and energetic manner of lifestyles.

Overtraining and its dangers.

Overtraining, also known as overtraining syndrome (OTS), takes region while there's an imbalance amongst schooling and healing. It's a country in which the frame does no longer have enough time to get higher efficiently from excessive workout, crucial to terrible bodily and psychological outcomes.

Overtraining poses severa risks and may have a unfavourable effect for your health and ordinary performance. Here are a number of the crucial detail dangers related to overtraining:

Physical Fatigue: Overtraining frequently outcomes in continual bodily fatigue, regardless of accurate sufficient rest. You also can feel continuously tired, slow, and lacking strength, making it hard to perform every day duties and sports.

Chapter 6: Supplements for Muscle Growth

Popular muscle-constructing dietary supplements are significantly used by people searching for to enhance their strength, muscle size, and commonplace athletic overall performance. These dietary supplements can supplement a nicely-balanced weight loss plan and a structured exercising software program application. Here, we are going to speak about of the maximum popular and properly-researched muscle-building dietary dietary supplements: protein and creatine.

1. Protein Supplements:

Protein is an essential macronutrient that plays a essential characteristic in muscle restore, growth, and regular restoration. Protein dietary supplements are convenient belongings of awesome protein and can be in particular useful for those who war to fulfill their protein wishes thru entire components by myself.

Types of Protein Supplements:

Whey Protein: Derived from milk, whey protein is a quick-digesting protein supply rich in important amino acids. It's first-rate for put up-workout restoration and is absorbed speedy via the body.

Casein Protein: Also derived from milk, casein protein is slow-digesting and offers a sustained launch of amino acids. It's suitable for midnight use or as a meal opportunity.

Plant-Based Proteins: Options like pea protein, rice protein, and hemp protein are appropriate for vegetarians and vegans. They also can have barely distinct amino acid profiles in assessment to animal-primarily based proteins.

How Protein Supplements Support Muscle Building:

Muscle Repair and Growth: Protein nutritional dietary supplements offer the amino acids vital for muscle restore and boom, especially after strenuous sporting activities.

Convenience: They offer a accessible manner to increase each day protein intake, in particular for humans with busy life.

Appetite Control: Protein can assist manipulate urge for food and promote feelings of fullness, which may be useful for those seeking to control their weight on the identical time as building muscle.

2. Creatine Supplements:

Creatine is a obviously taking vicinity compound decided in small portions in effective substances and synthesized thru the body. Creatine nutritional dietary supplements are seemed for his or her capability to enhance muscular electricity, power, and standard overall performance, making them a popular choice amongst athletes and electricity going for walks shoes.

How Creatine Supplements Support Muscle Building:

Improved ATP Production: Creatine allows growth the manufacturing of adenosine triphosphate (ATP), the number one strength deliver for muscle contractions at some stage in immoderate-depth, quick-length sports like weightlifting and sprinting.

Increased Muscle Hydration: Creatine can draw water into muscle cells, predominant to extended cell amount. This may additionally additionally make a contribution to muscle increase through cellular hydration.

Enhanced Muscle Recovery: Some studies suggests that creatine may moreover additionally lessen muscle harm and inflammation, probable helping in healing.

Greater Workout Intensity: Creatine supplementation can allow for extra intense sporting activities, that can help stimulate extra muscle boom through the years.

Usage Guidelines:

Loading Phase: Many human beings begin with a loading section, taking round 20 grams of creatine in step with day (split into 4 doses) for about each week, accompanied with the useful resource of a renovation segment of 3-five grams in step with day.

Timing: Creatine monohydrate is the most researched form and may be taken at any time of the day. Some select to take it placed up-workout for higher absorption.

Hydration: Ensure proper enough hydration whilst the use of creatine dietary nutritional dietary supplements to prevent any capability thing outcomes like cramping.

Important Considerations:

Individual Response: Not anybody responds to creatine in the equal manner. Some humans revel in massive blessings, at the same time as others may additionally moreover have a greater modest response.

Safety: Creatine is typically taken into consideration steady at the identical time as used as directed. However, talk over with a healthcare expert earlier than beginning any supplement habitual, in particular when you have underlying fitness situations.

Purity: Choose first rate producers that provide super, pure dietary dietary supplements with minimal additives.

While protein and creatine nutritional dietary supplements can be valuable device for muscle building, it is crucial to don't forget that they will be dietary dietary supplements, now not substitutes for a balanced eating regimen. Whole components want to stay the foundation of your nutritional intake. Additionally, consulting with a healthcare professional or registered dietitian earlier than starting any supplementation software is normally encouraged to make sure that it aligns at the facet of your individual health and health desires.

Benefits, risks, and tips for complement use.

Supplement use can offer blessings even as used as it must be, however it is crucial to be aware of ability dangers and observe suggestions to ensure consistent and effective supplementation. Here are the blessings, dangers, and hints for supplement use:

Benefits of Supplement Use:

Filling Nutritional Gaps: Supplements can help fill nutritional gaps while it's far hard to get all critical nutrients from meals on my own, at the side of for humans with specific nutritional rules or deficiencies.

Enhanced Athletic Performance: Certain nutritional nutritional supplements, like creatine and caffeine, were proven to improve athletic overall performance, power, and endurance.

Muscle Recovery and Growth: Protein dietary dietary supplements can useful resource in muscle recovery and increase, specially even as ate up after immoderate bodily video games.

Improved Health: Some nutritional nutritional dietary supplements, like omega-3 fatty acids, vitamins, and minerals, have confirmed health advantages, which consist of assisting coronary coronary heart fitness, lowering infection, and strengthening the immune device.

Weight Management: Supplements like fiber, inexperienced tea extract, and fine urge for food suppressants also can moreover assist in weight management and urge for food manage.

Risks of Supplement Use:

Lack of Regulation: The complement agency is a good deal less regulated than prescribed drugs, because of this that product best and safety can range appreciably among producers. Some dietary nutritional dietary supplements may additionally contain impurities or inaccurately categorised components.

Interactions with Medications: Certain dietary dietary supplements can have interaction with prescription drugs, probable reducing their effectiveness or inflicting negative effects. Always speak with a healthcare expert in advance than along with nutritional dietary supplements to your habitual, particularly in case you're taking drugs.

Overdosing: Excessive consumption of fantastic nutrients and minerals can result in toxicity, in all likelihood causing bad fitness outcomes. Follow advocated dosages and avoid taking multiple nutritional dietary supplements with the equal vitamins until cautioned by means of using a healthcare professional.

Misleading Claims: The complement industry is infamous for making unproven or exaggerated claims. Be cautious of dietary supplements promising marvelous results, and look for products with scientific backing.

Wasted Money: In some times, dietary nutritional dietary supplements might not provide critical advantages, principal to wasted coins and unhappiness.

Guidelines for Safe and Effective Supplement Use:

Consult a Healthcare Professional: Before starting any supplement routine, speak with a healthcare expert or registered dietitian. They can help you make a decision whether or not dietary supplements are vital, based totally mostly on your person health and dietary needs.

Choose Reputable Brands: Select nutritional dietary supplements from legitimate producers that adhere to right manufacturing practices (GMP). Look for zero.33-party finding out and certification to verify product first-class and purity.

Follow Recommended Dosages: Always study the advocated dosages and usage recommendations supplied at the complement label or as recommended via a healthcare expert.

Read Labels Carefully: Check complement labels for capability allergens, additives, fillers, and inactive materials that won't align together with your nutritional choices or sensitivities.

Avoid Mega-Dosing: Avoid excessive or mega-dosing of vitamins and minerals besides in particular recommended with the aid of a healthcare expert. More isn't normally higher and may on occasion be harmful.

Consider Food First: Strive to fulfill your nutritional needs via a balanced food regimen rich in complete meals. Supplements must supplement, now not replace, wholesome ingesting behavior.

Monitor Your Health: Keep song of approaches supplements have an effect for your fitness, and be aware about any modifications inside the way you enjoy. If you experience destructive results, prevent use and are looking for advice from a healthcare expert.

Be Cautious with Specialty Supplements: Be specially careful with location of know-how nutritional dietary supplements, weight loss tablets, and herbal remedies. These often lack rigorous medical proof and might have undisclosed risks.

Understand Your Goals: Determine your unique dreams for complement use, whether or not or now not it's far filling a nutritional gap, enhancing athletic everyday normal overall performance, or addressing a health hassle. This will guide your complement selections.

Regularly Reevaluate: Periodically reconsider the want for dietary dietary supplements in session with a healthcare professional. Your dietary dreams may also trade over time.

In summary, while nutritional supplements can provide benefits, in addition they deliver dangers if not used as it have to be. Consulting with a healthcare professional, selecting reliable products, and adhering to recommended dosages are vital practices for secure and effective complement use. Whole components ought to live the number one supply of nutrients in a balanced weight loss plan.

The position of nutritional dietary dietary supplements in a balanced healthy eating plan.

Supplements play a supportive feature in a balanced weight-reduction plan with the aid of assisting to fill nutritional gaps and deal with particular nutritional desires. While they're not an alternative to entire meals, dietary supplements can be valuable in top notch conditions. Here's the location of nutritional supplements in a balanced diet:

Filling Nutritional Gaps: Even with a nicely-rounded weight loss plan, it can be difficult to continuously meet all of your dietary desires from meals by myself. Supplements can provide vital nutrients, minerals, and special vitamins that can be missing to your food regimen due to factors like nutritional policies, meals hypersensitive reactions, or inadequate consumption of certain nutrients.

Addressing Specific Deficiencies: Supplements are often used to deal with identified nutrient deficiencies identified thru blood exams or clinical checks. Common deficiencies embody diet D, diet B12, iron, and calcium. In such instances, nutritional dietary supplements can help correct the deficiency and save you related health issues.

Enhancing Athletic Performance: Athletes and energetic people also can moreover use nutritional dietary supplements like protein, creatine, and branched-chain amino acids (BCAAs) to help muscle recovery, beautify power, and enhance endurance. These nutritional supplements can supplement a nicely-established training software and sell better exercise overall overall performance.

Supporting Overall Health: Certain nutritional dietary supplements, along side omega-3 fatty acids (placed in fish oil), can provide health advantages like decreasing contamination, supporting coronary coronary coronary heart health, and improving cognitive characteristic. These nutritional supplements may be encouraged thru healthcare experts to address particular health issues.

Convenience and Accessibility: In a few situations, dietary supplements can offer a handy and accessible manner to accumulate unique vitamins, specially at the same time as entire elements are not effects to be had or realistic. For example, protein powder may be a accessible choice submit-workout even as complete food resources aren't on hand.

Targeted Nutrient Intake: Supplements may be used for targeted nutrient consumption in the course of specific life tiers, together with pregnancy and breastfeeding. Prenatal nutrients, as an instance, offer vital nutrients like folic acid and iron to assist the fitness of every the mom and the developing fetus.

Dietary Preferences and Restrictions: Individuals with nutritional options or rules (e.G., vegetarians, vegans) may additionally moreover use dietary supplements to make certain they're assembly their nutrient desires. For instance, vegans can also take vitamins B12 dietary supplements because of the fact this nutrient is commonly positioned in animal-derived food.

It's essential to examine that dietary dietary supplements need to be used strategically and in consultation with a healthcare expert or registered dietitian. While they may be useful, taking immoderate or useless dietary dietary supplements can result in fitness dangers and imbalances.

A balanced diet, which encompass some of complete meals, ought to continuously shape the foundation of your nutritional intake. Whole substances provide a massive spectrum of vitamins, fiber, and distinct beneficial compounds that nutritional supplements can not reflect. By combining a balanced diet with thoughtful and sensible supplement use, you could optimize your dietary intake and aid regular health and nicely-being.

Chapter 7: Tracking Progress

Monitoring and measuring muscle and strength gains is crucial for monitoring progress, adjusting your schooling software program, and staying stimulated. Here are a few effective strategies and techniques to screen and diploma your income:

1. Keep a Workout Journal:

Maintain an extensive exercising magazine to file your training schooling. Include the subsequent statistics:

Date of the workout.

Exercises finished.

Sets and repetitions for every exercising.

Weight or resistance used.

Rest intervals among devices.

Notes on how you felt sooner or later of the exercise, together with electricity tiers, muscle pain, or any issues with form or method.

Reviewing your exercising magazine over the years will allow you to pick out out tendencies, song improvements, and observe areas that might need hobby.

2. Measure Strength Progress:

Strength profits are a number one indicator of muscle development. To degree power gains correctly:

Regularly perform energy exams for key physical video games. This should comprise one-repetition most (1RM) checks or attempting out your 5RM (the most weight you could deliver for 5 repetitions) for compound sports sports like bench press, squat, and deadlift.

Track modifications in the amount of weight you may increase for a specific range of repetitions (e.G., going from lifting one hundred thirty 5 pounds for 5 reps to a hundred and fifty five pounds for 5 reps shows improvement).

Use a schooling app or spreadsheet to record and graph your electricity profits through the years. Many apps can automatically calculate your estimated 1RM based totally on your units and reps.

3. Take Progress Photos:

Visual improvement can be motivating and help you display muscle gains. Take regular pics from taken into consideration one of a type angles in ordinary lighting fixtures to have a study changes in muscle definition, length, and everyday body.

Aim for constant intervals, consisting of every 4-8 weeks, to seize sizable adjustments.

Ensure ordinary conditions, much like the identical time of day, lights, and digital digicam setup, to make comparisons correct.

four. Measure Body Measurements:

Take measurements of key frame elements using a tape degree. Common areas to degree encompass:

Chest (at the nipple line).

Waist (at the narrowest point).

Hips (at the widest point).

Thighs (mid-thigh).

Biceps (on the midpoint).

Keep a report of those measurements and tune modifications through the years. While changes in frame measurements won't without a doubt replicate muscle profits (they may be stimulated via manner of the use of fat loss or advantage), they provide valuable insights into your improvement.

5. Use Body Composition Assessments:

Body composition tests, which include skinfold measurements or bioelectrical impedance assessment (BIA), can provide insights into modifications in muscle and fat mass. These assessments are typically greater correct than relying totally on weight measurements.

Consult a fitness professional or registered dietitian for correct and steady body composition measurements.

6. Assess Performance Metrics:

In addition to strength checks, undergo in thoughts tracking one in all a type standard overall performance metrics relevant on your health desires, which encompass:

Endurance (e.G., monitoring your 5K run time or the quantity of push-usayou may additionally want to do).

Power (e.G., vertical soar pinnacle or dash velocity).

Functional fitness checks (e.G., the capacity to carry out bodyweight sporting sports like pull-u.S.A.Or dips).

These metrics will let you gauge improvements in well-known fitness and athleticism.

7. Be Patient and Realistic:

Remember that muscle and energy earnings take time. Be affected man or woman and hold sensible expectations. Gains may not be linear, and there is probably durations of plateau. Consistency, proper vitamins, and true sufficient relaxation are key to lengthy-term improvement.

eight. Consult a Fitness Professional:

If you are uncertain approximately a way to track progress or have a look at your earnings as it need to be, bear in mind jogging with an authorized non-public trainer or fitness expert. They can provide steering, carry out assessments, and tailor your utility for your desires.

Regularly monitoring and measuring your muscle and electricity profits no longer most effective allows you live heading in the right direction but moreover permits you to regulate your schooling and vitamins techniques for persisted improvement and achievement.

Keeping exercise journals and logs.

Keeping exercise journals and logs is a precious exercise for truly everyone pursuing fitness desires, whether it's miles building muscle, dropping weight, enhancing staying power, or enhancing not unusual health. These statistics assist you tune improvement, live induced, and make informed selections approximately your training and nutrition. Here's a way to correctly preserve exercising journals and logs:

1. Choose a Format:

There are numerous codecs for exercising journals and logs, and you could select one which fits your alternatives:

Physical Journal/Notebook: A conventional pocket ebook or mag in which you can write down your exercise workouts using pen and paper.

Digital Apps: Many health apps and internet sites provide exercise tracking features. These apps frequently provide delivered benefits, which incorporates automated calculation of your education extent, development graphs, and the capacity to set reminders.

Spreadsheet: Create a workout log using spreadsheet software program like Microsoft Excel or Google Sheets. This allows for personalisation and easy information evaluation.

Online Platforms: Some on line health systems offer workout logging and monitoring abilties. You can log your workout workouts, percent them with others, and get admission to them from any tool with an internet connection.

2. Record Relevant Details:

Your exercise magazine have to embody important info to song improvement efficaciously:

Date: Record the date of every exercising to create a timeline of your training.

Exercises: List the physical video games you achieved in the end of your exercise. Include compound movements (e.G., bench press, squats) and isolation sporting occasions (e.G., bicep curls, leg extensions).

Sets and Repetitions: Specify the style of gadgets and repetitions for every exercising. For instance, three units of 10 reps.

Weights or Resistance: Note the quantity of weight lifted or the resistance used. This allows you track strength profits.

Rest Periods: Record the duration of rest intervals between gadgets and bodily video games.

Intensity or Difficulty: Use a score scale or notes to give an explanation for the intensity or trouble of your workout. This let you discover dispositions to your overall performance.

Notes: Include any applicable notes approximately your workout, which includes the manner you felt, changes made, or any stressful conditions encountered.

3. Set Clear Goals:

Establish unique, measurable goals that align together together with your fitness dreams. Whether you intention to growth power, construct muscle, lose weight, or beautify staying electricity, having clean desires will deliver your exercise physical activities purpose and direction.

4. Track Progress:

Consistently file your bodily sports and periodically assessment your magazine to song progress. Look for tendencies, upgrades, or regions wherein you could need changes.

Chapter 8: Common Mistakes and How to Avoid Them

Muscle constructing is a aim that many humans pursue, but it isn't unusual to make mistakes alongside the way. Identifying and addressing the ones commonplace mistakes is important to attaining powerful and sustainable muscle growth. Here are a few often going on errors in muscle constructing and the way to deal with them:

1. Inadequate Nutrition:

Mistake: Not ingesting sufficient electricity, protein, or vital vitamins to guide muscle boom.

Solution:

Calculate your each day caloric desires, at the side of a surplus of energy to manual muscle boom (typically 250-500 energy above maintenance).

Prioritize protein intake, aiming for 1.2 to two.2 grams of protein constant with kilogram of frame weight.

Include an entire lot of nutrient-dense additives on your eating regimen, which embody lean meats, fish, complete grains, culmination, greens, and healthy fat.

2. Neglecting Progressive Overload:

Mistake: Sticking with the same weight or resistance stages in your carrying activities without regularly developing them.

Solution:

Regularly boom the burden, reps, or depth of your bodily video games to mission your muscle tissues.

Follow a set up education software that consists of revolutionary overload necessities.

3. Overtraining:

Mistake: Training too frequently or intensely with out permitting sufficient time for recuperation.

Solution:

Prioritize rest and recuperation, along with proper sleep, nutrients, and active recovery techniques (e.G., stretching, foam rolling).

Ensure that your exercise utility consists of pinnacle enough relaxation days and avoids immoderate quantity.

four. Lack of Variation:

Mistake: Doing the identical bodily video video games and workout exercises for an extended length, most crucial to plateaus.

Solution:

Incorporate variety into your workouts with the resource of changing sports activities, rep ranges, and training techniques.

Periodize your education utility to embody degrees of different intensities and focuses (e.G., energy, hypertrophy, patience).

5. Poor Form and Technique:

Mistake: Using mistaken shape and method, that would motive injuries and decrease muscle engagement.

Solution:

Focus on right workout shape and approach. Consider running with a certified personal instructor to make certain you are using correct shape.

Use lighter weights whilst studying new bodily sports or whilst form starts offevolved to go to pot due to fatigue.

6. Inadequate Warm-Up and Mobility Work:

Mistake: Skipping warmth-up and mobility sports activities, which can restrict your form of motion and boom the chance of damage.

Solution:

Incorporate a radical warmness-up ordinary that consists of dynamic stretching and mobility bodily sports.

Pay interest to joint fitness and flexibility to make sure entire style of motion in the route of sports activities.

7. Neglecting Recovery and Sleep:

Mistake: Not giving your body enough time to get better amongst physical video games and now not getting sufficient sleep.

Solution:

Prioritize sleep and goal for 7-9 hours of tremendous sleep everyday with night time.

Schedule rest days and lively recovery days as part of your schooling software program.

eight. Overreliance on Supplements:

Mistake: Relying too closely on nutritional supplements with out addressing diet plan and education basics.

Solution:

Use dietary supplements as a complement to a properly-balanced food regimen and education program, no longer as an opportunity.

Consult with a healthcare professional or registered dietitian to decide if dietary dietary supplements are essential based totally to your particular desires.

nine. Impatience:

Mistake: Expecting rapid consequences and becoming discouraged even as development is slower than predicted.

Solution:

Understand that muscle constructing is a slow manner that takes time.

Focus on regular try and have amusing small victories along the manner to maintain motivation.

10. Inconsistent Training:

Mistake: Skipping exercise exercises or following an inconsistent education agenda.

Solution:

Establish a steady training routine and stick with it as closely as possible.

Prioritize workouts and make them a non-negotiable a part of a while table.

Identifying and addressing those not unusual mistakes in muscle constructing will allow you to make extra green development and reduce the danger of damage. Remember that staying strength and a holistic technique to education, vitamins, and recuperation are key to reaching your muscle-constructing desires very well and correctly.

Tips for stopping injuries.

Preventing injuries is important for keeping a regular and effective health routine. Here are a few recommendations that will help you reduce the threat of injuries sooner or later of exercise:

1. Warm-Up Adequately:

Start your exercising with a proper warmth-as a good deal as put together your body for brought excessive hobby. A warmness-up need to include moderate aerobic workout (e.G., jogging or leaping jacks) and dynamic stretching to boom blood drift and unfasten muscle tissues and joints.

2. Use Proper Form and Technique:

Perform sports with accurate shape and approach. Poor shape can reason overuse accidents, strains, and sprains. If you're unsure approximately your form, recollect operating with a certified private teacher or health professional.

three. Progress Gradually:

Avoid overexerting your self thru progressing grade by grade in phrases of weight, depth, and volume. Gradual improvement allows your frame to evolve and decreases the chance of sudden injuries.

4. Listen to Your Body:

Pay hobby on your frame's indicators. If you revel in pain or pain past normal muscle ache, save you the exercising and affirm the problem. Pushing thru pain can bring about injuries.

5. Balance Your Workouts:

Include plenty of sporting sports activities that focus on top notch muscle corporations to prevent overuse accidents. Balanced sports additionally assist save you muscle imbalances, that would bring about accidents.

6. Incorporate Rest Days:

Rest days are vital for healing. Overtraining can purpose fatigue and boom the chance of accidents. Schedule normal relaxation days and prioritize sleep to allow your body to restore and rejuvenate.

7. Use Appropriate Footwear:

Wear proper athletic shoes that offer manual and cushioning on your precise hobby. Ill-becoming or worn-out footwear can growth the chance of foot and ankle injuries.

eight. Hydrate and Maintain Proper Nutrition:

Stay hydrated in advance than, during, and after workout to save you dehydration, that can purpose muscle cramps and warmth-associated troubles. Proper vitamins is also vital for normal fitness and damage prevention.

nine. Incorporate Flexibility and Mobility Work:

Include flexibility and mobility bodily activities on your recurring to beautify joint style of movement and reduce the threat of strains and sprains. Regular stretching can help preserve flexibility.

10. Warm Down After Exercise:

After your workout, carry out static stretching and deep respiration carrying sports to regularly cool down and reduce muscle anxiety. This can resource in recuperation and reduce post-workout soreness.

11. Cross-Train:

Mix up your exercise workout routines with wonderful styles of bodily sports activities and sports. Cross-education can reduce the hazard of overuse injuries associated with repetitive motions.

12. Stay Mindful During Exercise:

Maintain recognition and mindfulness in some unspecified time within the destiny of your exercising exercises. Avoid distractions that could bring about horrible shape or injuries.

13. Know Your Limits:

While it's far crucial to mission yourself, it's far similarly essential to understand your limits. Pushing too difficult, specifically while fatigued, can bring about accidents. Be sensible about your fitness diploma.

14. Seek Professional Guidance:

If you are new to exercising or have specific fitness worries, talk over with a healthcare professional or health expert in advance than beginning a new health software. They can provide steering tailored on your character goals.

15. Consider Strength Training:

Strength education can assist enhance joint balance and decrease the danger of accidents. Incorporate resistance physical video games that target most critical muscle agencies.

Remember that accidents can still stand up however taking precautions. If you do revel in an harm, are seeking out set off scientific hobby and observe a rehabilitation plan to ensure a consistent and effective healing. Prioritizing damage prevention thru the ones guidelines will let you maintain a healthful and damage-unfastened health adventure.

Managing plateaus and setbacks.

Experiencing plateaus and setbacks is a common a part of any fitness adventure, but the manner you manipulate and triumph over them can considerably effect your prolonged-term improvement and motivation. Here are a few techniques for coping with plateaus and setbacks successfully:

1. Reevaluate Your Goals:

When you hit a plateau or come across a setback, take a step lower lower back and reconsider your dreams. Are they despite the fact that applicable and possible? Adjust your desires if vital to stay inspired and focused.

2. Change Your Routine:

Plateaus regularly upward push up whilst your body becomes familiar with a specific exercising ordinary. Change things up thru introducing new physical video video games, converting the order of your workout exercises, or adjusting the intensity and volume. This alternate can stimulate particular muscle businesses and break the plateau.

three. Periodize Your Training:

Implement a periodization plan in your exercise regular. Periodization involves cycling via ranges of severa schooling intensities and focuses, which include power, hypertrophy, and patience. This approach permits save you overtraining and continues your workouts clean.

four. Focus on Nutrition:

Review your nutrients plan and make sure you're assembly your calorie and macronutrient needs. A nutritionist or registered dietitian will permit you to extremely good-track your weight loss program to help your desires. Consider tracking your food intake for a period to choose out regions for development.

five. Rest and Recovery:

Adequate rest and recuperation are critical for progress. Ensure you are becoming enough brilliant sleep, scheduling relaxation days into your ordinary, and strolling towards lively restoration strategies like stretching and foam rolling.

Chapter 9: Staying Motivated and Sustaining Gains

Maintaining lengthy-term dedication to muscle training may be difficult, but with the right techniques, you can live advocated and committed on your fitness goals over the prolonged haul. Here are some powerful strategies for ensuring your determination remains strong:

1. Define Clear and Specific Goals:

Set smooth, specific, and measurable fitness goals. Knowing what you're running toward gives a revel in of purpose and route. Break your lengthy-time period goals into smaller, achievable milestones to have fun along the way.

2. Find Intrinsic Motivation:

Identify and interest on internal motivations for education, including advanced fitness, extended electricity, and a experience of achievement. Intrinsic motivation is extra sustainable than outdoor factors like look or opposition.

three. Create a Consistent Routine:

Establish a workout everyday that fits your way of lifestyles and opportunities. Choose physical games and sports activities activities you revel in and discover a exercise time desk that you can realistically maintain. Consistency is high to prolonged-term achievement.

four. Embrace Variety and Progression:

Incorporate range into your exercises to prevent boredom and plateaus. Try new sports sports, schooling techniques, and stressful situations to maintain topics easy and exciting. Always intention to improvement in a few manner, whether or not it's miles developing weight, reps, or intensity.

five. Track Your Progress:

Keep an intensive exercising mag to music your development over the years. Seeing enhancements in electricity, patience, or muscle increase can be fairly motivating. Use seen aids like pix or measurements to file your journey.

6. Find Accountability:

Workout with a chum, be a part of a health company, or rent a non-public teacher. Having someone to percentage your health journey with and maintain you responsible can enhance motivation and consistency.

7. Reward Yourself:

Celebrate your achievements and milestones with rewards. Treat your self even as you attain a specific intention or keep on together with your education plan usually. Rewards can offer notable reinforcement.

8. Prioritize Recovery:

Recognize the significance of rest and healing. Overtraining can motive burnout and injuries.

Incorporate relaxation days into your normal and prioritize sleep and right vitamins for remaining recovery.

9. Stay Educated:

Continuously train yourself approximately exercising, nutrients, and education necessities. Understanding the "why" and "how" in the back of your workout exercises can deepen your dedication and exuberance.

10. Set New Challenges:

Regularly set new health demanding conditions to keep your physical video games thrilling. These disturbing situations can embody attempting a present day exercise, competing in an event, or studying a tough exercise.

eleven. Practice Mindfulness:

Be present sooner or later of your exercise physical activities and exercise mindfulness. Focusing at the mind-frame connection can enhance your education revel in and decorate technique.

12. Adapt to Life Changes:

Life is dynamic, and commitments alternate. Be bendy in adjusting your education routine to house lifestyles occasions, artwork, and circle of relatives responsibilities. Finding a balance is important for long-time period willpower.

thirteen. Renew Your Motivation:

Periodically re-look at your desires and motivations. Life activities and priorities also can evolve, so it is vital to renew your dedication as wished.

14. Seek Professional Guidance:

Consider strolling with a licensed personal trainer or health educate. They can provide information, create tailor-made packages, and offer assist to preserve you on the proper tune.

15. Enjoy the Journey:

Lastly, bear in thoughts to revel in the adventure itself. Fitness is a lifelong pursuit, and the technique can be as profitable because of the reality the effects. Celebrate your development and consist of the disturbing situations.

Maintaining lengthy-time period dedication to muscle education requires a mixture of strength of will, motivation, and versatility. By incorporating the ones strategies into your fitness journey, you will be higher prepared to live dedicated and reap your muscle schooling dreams over the long run.

Setting new goals and demanding situations.

Setting new desires and annoying conditions is a essential factor of private growth, whether or not or no longer or now not it's miles within the realm of fitness, career, or personal improvement. Here's a step-through-step guide on a way to set new dreams and demanding situations effectively:

1. Reflect on Your Current Situation:

Take a while to mirror to your cutting-edge conditions and achievements. Consider what you have got finished to this point and in that you stand almost about your lengthy-time period goals. This self-assessment allows you choose out areas for improvement and new instructions to find out.

2. Define Your Values and Priorities:

Clarify your values and priorities in life. What sincerely subjects to you? Understanding your middle values will assist you align your desires and demanding situations with what is most huge to you. For example, if health and health are crucial values, setting fitness-associated dreams can be a trouble.

3. Set SMART Goals:

Create goals which is probably Specific, Measurable, Achievable, Relevant, and Time-sure (SMART). SMART dreams offer clean route and a concrete plan for motion. For example, in region of a vague intention like "Get in form," a SMART intention is probably

"Lose 10 pounds in three months with the useful resource of exercise 3 times according to week and following a balanced food plan."

four. Consider Short-Term and Long-Term Goals:

Differentiate among brief-time period and prolonged-term desires. Short-term dreams are smaller, greater immediately objectives that make contributions in your extended-time period vision. For instance, a quick-term goal can be enhancing your weekly exercise consistency, even as the lengthy-time period aim may be engaging in a particular fitness milestone.

five. Challenge Yourself:

Set tough desires that push you out of your consolation region. A properly task should be ambitious however attainable with try to self-discipline. Stepping out of doors your comfort zone can purpose private growth and prolonged motivation.

6. Break Goals into Actionable Steps:

Break down your dreams into smaller, actionable steps or obligations. This makes them greater potential and plenty much less overwhelming. These smaller steps feature a roadmap to task your huge goals.

7. Prioritize and Sequence Your Goals:

Consider the collection in which you can pursue your desires. Some desires might also need to be completed earlier than others can be tackled. Prioritize your goals primarily based on their importance and relevance to your present day events.

eight. Set a Deadline:

Assign ultimate dates for your dreams and demanding situations. Having a time frame creates a feel of urgency and enables you live accountable. However, make certain your remaining dates are sensible and aligned with the complexity of the cause.

9. Monitor and Adjust:

Regularly display your improvement inside the course of your dreams. If you come upon boundaries or find that your priorities have shifted, be open to adjusting your desires or your technique to accomplishing them. Flexibility is critical to conform to changing sports.

10. Seek Support and Accountability:

Share your desires with a trusted buddy, member of the family, or mentor who can offer resource and maintain you responsible. Social obligation can encourage you to stay dedicated.

eleven. Stay Motivated and Positive:

Maintain your motivation with the resource of visualizing your success and focusing at the brilliant elements of pursuing your desires. Celebrate your achievements, irrespective of how small, and remind yourself of the advantages you may benefit from assignment them.

12. Embrace Failure as a Learning Opportunity:

Recognize that setbacks and disasters are a herbal part of pursuing worrying conditions. Rather than seeing them as barriers, view them as valuable studying opportunities that might inform your destiny efforts.

thirteen. Stay Consistent:

Consistency is fundamental to reaching your goals and overcoming traumatic situations. Make every day or weekly efforts, even though motivation wanes. The cumulative impact of regular motion is frequently what results in fulfillment.

14. Review and Adjust Regularly:

Periodically assessment your desires, have a look at your development, and regulate your method as wished. Life conditions exchange, and your goals want to adapt consequently.

Setting new dreams and annoying situations is a effective manner to pressure private growth and gather what topics maximum to you. By following those steps and preserving a proactive attitude, you may constantly set and gather significant targets in severa factors of your existence.

Celebrating successes and staying inspired.

Celebrating successes and staying inspired are crucial factors of keeping motivation and momentum to your adventure to benefit your dreams. Here are a few strategies to help you rejoice your successes and hold your notion alive:

1. Acknowledge and Reflect:

Take a 2d to acknowledge and reflect for your achievements, no matter how small or big they will be. Recognizing your successes permits assemble self guarantee and reinforces your willpower.

Chapter 10: Understanding Protein's Role

2.1 Explanation of protein's importance in muscle building

Protein is a important problem in muscle constructing, gambling a critical function in diverse physiological processes that make contributions to muscle increase and restore. Here's an evidence of protein's importance in muscle constructing:

1.   Muscle Protein Synthesis (MPS): Protein consists of amino acids, which might be the building blocks of muscle mass. When you interact in resistance training or distinctive sorts of workout, you create microscopic harm to muscle fibers. Protein intake stimulates muscle protein synthesis, the device through which the frame safety and rebuilds those damaged muscle fibers, making them stronger and massive.

2.   Amino Acid Profile: Proteins consist of diverse amino acids, a number of which may be essential and cannot be produced by way of manner of the frame. Consuming quite a

few protein resources guarantees that your frame gets all the critical amino acids essential for ideal muscle boom and restore.

three. Positive Nitrogen Balance: Nitrogen stability refers to the distinction among the amount of nitrogen taken in through protein and the quantity excreted. A high-quality nitrogen stability, in which more nitrogen is retained, is related to an anabolic (muscle-building) united states of america. Adequate protein intake lets in keep a exquisite nitrogen stability, assisting muscle boom.

4. Energy Source: While carbohydrates and fat are the number one resources of strength for the frame, protein can be used as an electricity supply whilst wanted, especially in the route of intervals of calorie deficit. This allows spare muscular tissues from being used for strength and preserves it for growth and restore.

5. Hormonal Regulation: Protein consumption affects the release of various hormones, which incorporates insulin and

boom hormone, which play important roles in muscle growth. Insulin allows go back and forth amino acids into cells, selling protein synthesis, while increase hormone stimulates ordinary tissue growth.

6.   Appetite Regulation: Protein has a satiating effect, which means it enables you revel in complete and happy. This can be beneficial for the ones looking to manage their body weight, as it can make a contribution to better urge for meals control and in all likelihood useful resource fats loss at the identical time as keeping muscle tissues.

7.   Muscle   Preservation   throughout Weight Loss: When aiming to shed kilos, making sure an appropriate enough protein consumption will become essential for maintaining lean muscle mass. This is crucial due to the reality dropping muscle corporations together with fats can avoid metabolism and make it extra hard to preserve weight loss.

eight. Recovery and Reduced Muscle Soreness: Protein intake placed up-workout aids inside the restoration technique via providing the vital building blocks for muscle restore. It also can help reduce muscle soreness, taking into consideration quicker and extra inexperienced recovery among workout physical games.

In precis, protein is crucial for muscle building as it offers the important amino acids, helps muscle protein synthesis, regulates hormones, and plays a vital function in everyday muscle fitness and feature. Including an ok quantity of exceptional protein on your diet is a key trouble in optimizing muscle growth and healing.

2.2 How a splendid deal protein ought to be consumed

The maximum dependable quantity of protein one have to eat is predicated upon on various factors, including person desires, age, gender, pastime degree, and established health. While the Recommended Dietary Allowance

(RDA) devices the minimal at 0.Eight grams of protein consistent with kilogram of frame weight for sedentary adults, those venture normal bodily interest, mainly muscle-constructing sports activities sports, can also benefit from a higher consumption within the type of 1.6 to two.2 grams in keeping with kilogram. It's crucial to look at that the ones are general pointers, and person protein desires can also moreover fluctuate based totally totally on elements like age, metabolism, and particular health dreams. Consulting with a healthcare expert or registered dietitian for customized advice tailor-made to person events is suggested. Distributing protein consumption lightly within the direction of the day is likewise key to helping muscle protein synthesis.

2.Three Healthy belongings of protein for muscle building

Certainly! There are numerous nutritious assets of protein that might assist muscle development. Here are a few alternatives:

Lean Meats: Opt for lean cuts of bird, turkey, red meat, and pork for extremely good protein with out more saturated fats.

Fish: Fatty fish like salmon, tuna, and mackerel no longer satisfactory provide protein but moreover provide omega-three fatty acids, that have more fitness blessings.

Eggs: Eggs function a entire protein supply, containing all crucial amino acids, and they are flexible in education.

Dairy Products: Greek yogurt, cottage cheese, and milk are rich in protein and provide delivered calcium for bone health.

Plant-Based Proteins: Legumes along facet beans, lentils, and chickpeas, along aspect tofu, tempeh, and edamame, are excellent plant-based protein belongings. Whole grains like quinoa furthermore make a contribution.

Nuts and Seeds: Almonds, peanuts, chia seeds, and pumpkin seeds not quality offer protein but additionally deliver wholesome fat and other vital nutrients.

Protein-Rich Vegetables: Broccoli, spinach, peas, and Brussels sprouts include a decent quantity of protein at the same time as contributing to not unusual nutrient consumption.

Protein Supplements: Whey protein, casein protein, and plant-based totally completely protein powders can be accessible for meeting protein needs, specifically for people with better necessities.

Lean Protein Snacks: Choose jerky without excessive components, protein bars with limited sugar, and roasted chickpeas as healthy, on-the-glide protein alternatives.

Seitan: This is a immoderate-protein meat substitute made from gluten (wheat protein), often embraced in vegetarian and vegan diets.

Remember, keeping a balanced diet that includes plenty of protein belongings guarantees a whole intake of vital amino acids and distinctive essential nutrients for wellknown health and muscle building. Consulting with a nutritionist or healthcare expert can help tailor your protein intake to your particular dreams and nutritional alternatives.

Building a Nutrition Plan for Muscle Building

three.1 Macronutrients and their significance Certainly! Macronutrients are important vitamins the body desires in larger portions to feature efficiently. They feature the number one property of energy and assist diverse physiological techniques. The three primary macronutrients—carbohydrates, proteins, and fat—each have particular roles.

1. Carbohydrates:

Significance: Carbohydrates are the primary electricity supply for the body. They destroy down into glucose, offering power for every day sports and maintaining brain characteristic. Carbs are saved as glycogen in muscle tissue and the liver for later use all through exercising or durations of low food consumption.

2.   Proteins:

Importance: Proteins play a crucial position in building and repairing tissues. Composed of amino acids, they contribute to muscle improvement, immune characteristic, enzyme manufacturing, and the protection of pores and pores and pores and skin, hair, and nails. Proteins are also concerned in the manufacturing of hormones and particular signaling molecules.

3.   Fats:

Importance: Fats are a focused electricity supply and are essential for soaking up fats-soluble nutrients (A, D, E, K). They offer insulation, guard organs, and make contributions to mobile form. Essential fatty acids, like omega-3 and omega-6, need to be obtained from the healthy dietweight-reduction plan because the body can't produce them.

In summary:

Energy Production: Carbohydrates and fats feature primary electricity property, with carbohydrates being the body's preferred and consequences available supply.

Tissue Repair and Growth: Proteins are critical for repairing and building tissues, playing a pivotal feature in muscle development and common bodily form.

Metabolic Functions: Each macronutrient has fantastic metabolic functions. Carbohydrates regulate blood sugar, proteins help enzyme and hormone production, and fat make contributions to severa cell techniques.

Vital Nutrients: Macronutrients provide vital nutrients essential for the body's proper functioning, influencing popular fitness and nicely-being.

Achieving a balanced consumption of these macronutrients is important for maintaining a healthy and properly-rounded weight loss program. The precise proportions can also range primarily based totally on character desires, desires, and way of life factors. Emphasizing the intake of whole, nutrient-dense food is critical for quality fitness.

1.   Three.2 Meal planning for muscle constructing Determine Your Caloric Requirements:

Calculate your each day calorie dreams primarily based simply for your goals (protection, bulking, or slicing). This serves as a foundation for installing your macronutrient objectives.

2.   Establish Protein Intake:

Aim for a sufficient protein consumption, usually ranging from 1.6 to two.2 grams of protein constant with kilogram of frame weight. Include lean protein property like fowl, fish, lean beef, eggs, and plant-primarily based proteins together with tofu and legumes.

3.   Incorporate Carbohydrates:

Carbohydrates are crucial for presenting power, specially at some stage in severe exercising exercises. Opt for complicated carbohydrates like complete grains, brown rice, quinoa, sweet potatoes, and oats. These additionally make contributions fiber, supporting digestive fitness.

4. Include Healthy Fats:

Integrate assets of healthful fat inclusive of avocados, nuts, seeds, olive oil, and fatty fish. These fats sell fashionable fitness, useful aid in hormone production, and facilitate the absorption of fats-soluble vitamins.

five. Prioritize Post-Workout Nutrition:

Consume a publish-exercise meal or snack containing a mix of protein and carbohydrates to beneficial useful aid muscle healing and fill up glycogen shops. This must encompass a protein shake with fruit, Greek yogurt with berries, or a chook and quinoa bowl.

6. Spread Protein Intake Throughout the Day:

Distribute your protein intake frivolously at some point of meals to optimize muscle protein synthesis. Incorporate protein-wealthy snacks like Greek yogurt, cottage cheese, or protein bars among meals.

7. Include a Variety of Nutrient-Rich Foods:

Ensure your food encompass pretty a few colorful veggies and surrender quit result to provide nutrients and minerals. These make contributions antioxidants and assist normal health.

8. Stay Hydrated:

Maintain specific enough water consumption at some stage in the day to help common hydration and facilitate most suitable bodily functions, on the aspect of nutrient shipping and muscle recuperation.

9. Plan Ahead:

Prepare food and snacks in advance to avoid resorting to much less nutritious options at the same time as hungry. This may additionally contain batch cooking, portioning meals, and having healthful snacks with out trouble to be had.

10.   Consider Supplements:

If crucial, include dietary dietary dietary supplements like protein powder, creatine, and omega-three fatty acids to bridge nutritional gaps and assist muscle-building goals.

Remember, character goals variety, so it's far vital to alter your meal plan based totally on personal possibilities, nutritional guidelines, and your reaction to amazing meals. Seeking steerage from a registered dietitian or nutritionist can offer customized recommendation tailored in your particular desires and necessities.

Chapter 11: Training Techniques

4.1   Understanding   the   Correct   Form
Understanding the proper method for training your muscle tissues is vital for optimizing your exercise exercises and minimizing the risk of harm. Consider the ones crucial factors:

1.   Correct Form:

Emphasize preserving the right form in the course of each exercise to goal the intended muscle   companies   and   decrease   the probability of pressure or harm.

2.   Foundational Movements:

If you are new to a selected exercise, provoke with lighter weights or resistance. Master the important moves in advance than advancing to greater complicated versions.

3.   Complete Range of Motion:

Execute sporting activities via their complete type of movement to engage muscle tissues correctly   and   decorate   flexibility.   Avoid shortcuts or counting on momentum in the direction of weightlifting.

four.   Controlled Movements:

Focus on controlled actions at some point of each the muscle shortening (concentric) and extending (eccentric) ranges. Avoid abrupt or jerky motions that may result in damage.

five.   Mind-Muscle Connection:

Develop a connection amongst your mind and the targeted muscle in the course of each exercise.   This   intellectual   engagement enhances the efficiency of your exercising.

6.   Warm-Up:

Always perform an extensive heat-up in advance than task awesome resistance schooling. A right warm-up boosts blood glide, improves flexibility, and readies your body for the exercising.

7.   Progressive Overload:

Gradually boom workout depth to challenge your muscle agencies and stimulate boom. This development can also contain raising weights, repetitions, or resistance over time.

8.   Rest and Recovery:

Allow sufficient relaxation among devices and include relaxation days into your number one education utility. Adequate rest is important for muscle recovery and electricity enhancement.

nine.   Listening to Your Body:

Be privy to any ache or ache at some point of exercise exercises. If you experience sharp or continual pain, prevent and re-compare your form. Seek guidance from a fitness professional if important.

10.   Diverse Workouts:

Include numerous bodily video games for your habitual to aim splendid muscle companies, stopping overuse accidents and fostering balanced muscle improvement.

eleven.   Hydration:

Ensure right hydration for max useful muscle feature and favored normal performance. Dehydration can motive fatigue and increase damage dangers.

12.   Professional Guidance:

Consider partnering with a health trainer, especially if you're new to resistance education. They can offer path on proper shape, create a custom designed exercising plan, and screen your improvement.

Remember, prioritizing extraordinary over amount in your sporting activities contributes to prolonged-term fulfillment and a solid and inexperienced   muscle-constructing adventure.

four.1 Common Mistakes to Avoid

Certainly! Avoiding commonplace mistakes is vital for an powerful and solid muscle education adventure. Here are some key pitfalls to influence easy of:

Incorrect Form:

Using mistaken shape for the duration of physical games can result in injuries and restriction muscle activation. Prioritize correct shape over heavy weights.

Skipping Warm-Up:

Neglecting a proper heat-up will increase the threat of harm. Warm up your muscle mass with dynamic stretches and mild aerobic earlier than mission excessive resistance schooling.

Overtraining:

Excessive schooling without specific enough relaxation can reason fatigue, overuse accidents, and save you muscle recuperation. Allow for rest days and pay attention in your body.

Neglecting Compound Movements:

Focusing mostly on isolation sporting occasions and neglecting compound actions can limit primary muscle development.

Include pretty some sporting occasions in your routine.

Insufficient Variety:

Sticking to the same ordinary for too lengthy can purpose plateaus .

Ignoring Muscular Imbalances:

Neglecting imbalances in muscle power can cause horrific posture and increase the danger of injuries. Include sports sports that deal with imbalances.

Not Adjusting Resistance:

Failing to regularly boom resistance can restrict muscle boom. Gradually increase weights or resistance to provide an ongoing mission.

Inconsistent Training:

Inconsistency to your schooling ordinary can avert development. Stick to a ordinary time table to see sustained outcomes.

Insufficient Recovery:

Lack of proper healing, which consist of sleep and nutrients, can prevent muscle restore and increase. Prioritize recovery to maximise education blessings.

Ignoring Nutrition:

Nutrition performs a vital role in muscle building. Ensure you're ingesting sufficient protein, carbohydrates, and healthy fat to beneficial aid your training desires.

Over-Reliance on Machines:

While machines have their vicinity, relying truely on them can also forget stabilization muscular tissues. Incorporate loose weights and frame weight carrying occasions for a balanced approach.

Lack of Goal Setting:

Training with out smooth dreams can bring about aimless bodily games. Set precise, measurable goals to guide your training and track development.

Excessive Cardio:

Excessive cardiovascular exercise without properly sufficient power schooling can bring about muscle loss. Find a stability among aerobic and resistance education.

Not Listening to Your Body:

Ignoring pain or pushing thru injuries can get worse situations. Listen to your frame, alter bodily video video games if wanted, and are trying to find for expert recommendation for chronic issues.

Poor Hydration:

Inadequate hydration can have an effect on common performance and recuperation. Stay hydrated to guide regular muscle function.

By being privy to the ones common errors, you can enhance the effectiveness of your muscle education and reduce the risk of setbacks or accidents.

Chapter 12: Exercise Routine for Muscle Building

5.1. Comprehensive list of sporting occasions for muscle constructing Upper Body:

1.   Chest:

Perform Bench Press

Engage in Dumbbell Flyes

Include Push-Ups on your ordinary

2.   Back:

Execute Deadlifts

Incorporate Bent Over Rows

Do Lat Pulldowns

three. Shoulders:

Practice Military Press

Perform Lateral Raises

Include Face Pulls

4.   Arms:

Execute Bicep Curls

Engage in Tricep Dips

Include Hammer Curls

Lower Body:

Quads:

Perform Squats (each Back and Front)

Use the Leg Press device

Include Lunges for your ordinary

Hamstrings:

Execute Deadlifts (particularly Romanian)

Incorporate Leg Curls

Do Good Mornings

Glutes:

Engage in Hip Thrusts

Execute Glute Bridges

Include Bulgarian Split Squats

1. Calves:

Perform Standing Calf Raises

Engage in Seated Calf Raises

Include Calf Press on the Leg Press Machine

Core:

1. Abs:

Practice Planks

Engage in Russian Twists

Include Hanging Leg Raises

2. Obliques:

Execute Side Planks

Practice Woodchoppers

Engage in Bicycle Crunches

Remember to initiate with a weight that demanding situations you at the same time as retaining right form. Gradually growth the burden as your energy improves. Prioritize amazing shape over lifting heavier weights. Also, make sure a proper warmth-up in advance than beginning and a cool down in some time.

5.2 Proper techniques for specific bodily video games

Bench Press:

Lie in your lower back on a flat bench.

Grasp the bar with a grip barely wider than your shoulders.

Lower the bar to your chest, retaining a ninety-degree mind-set collectively at the side of your elbows.

Push the bar upward to the begin characteristic.

Chapter 13: The Importance of Cardiovascular Health in Men

Your coronary coronary heart fitness is essential to normal right fitness. It's answerable for pumping nutrient-rich blood for the duration of your body, it sources oxygen on the same time as casting off pollutants and waste. Lowered threat of sickness. Aerobic exercising reduces your threat of developing many ailments, which includes:

Better strength and stamina. Your coronary heart and lungs gets stronger as you exercise

A more active immune system

Managed weight

Stronger bones

Better temper

Lower blood pressure

Improve blood flow

Improve workout overall performance

Lower cholesterol

Decrease threat of coronary coronary heart ailment, stroke and diabetes

Promote different coronary coronary heart-healthy conduct

6.2 Explanation of cardiovascular Cardiovascular fitness relates to the general state of affairs of the coronary coronary heart and blood vessels, collectively called the cardiovascular tool. This tool is answerable for circulating blood, oxygen, and vitamins for the duration of the frame. Preserving most exceptional cardiovascular fitness is important for common properly-being and durability. Here are key elements and elements related to cardiovascular health:

Heart Well-being:

The coronary coronary heart, a muscular organ, propels blood at some stage in the frame.

Cardiovascular health includes the powerful functioning of the coronary coronary heart to distribute oxygen and vitamins to all cells.

Blood Vessels:

Arteries, veins, and capillaries represent the network of blood vessels.

Arteries delivery oxygenated blood away from the coronary coronary heart, on the identical time as veins pass lower back deoxygenated blood to the coronary coronary heart.

Capillaries hyperlink arteries and veins, facilitating the change of vitamins and oxygen with tissues.

Blood Pressure:

Blood pressure denotes the pressure of blood in competition to arterial partitions.

Elevated blood pressure (high blood stress) can pressure the coronary coronary heart and make a contribution to numerous cardiovascular issues.

Cholesterol Levels:

Cholesterol, a fatty substance inside the blood, calls for a healthful stability.

Elevated tiers of LDL (low-density lipoprotein) ldl ldl cholesterol, frequently termed "horrible" ldl ldl ldl cholesterol, can cause arterial plaque accumulation.

Exercise and Physical Activity:

Regular exercise fortifies the coronary heart, enhances blood stream, and aids in keeping a healthy weight.

Aerobic sports, together with strolling, walking, and biking, are specifically satisfactory for cardiovascular fitness.

Healthy Diet:

A balanced and coronary heart-exceptional food plan encompasses cease end end result, greens, complete grains, lean proteins, and coffee-fats dairy.

Limiting saturated and trans fats, sodium, and taken sugars is crucial for cardiovascular properly-being.

Avoiding Smoking and Moderating Alcohol Intake:

Smoking harms blood vessels and contributes to cardiovascular disorder.

Excessive alcohol consumption can also adversely have an impact on the cardiovascular machine.

Stress Management:

Prolonged strain can impact cardiovascular health. Practices like meditation or deep respiratory assist alleviate strain.

Regular Health Checkups:

Routine examinations with healthcare experts beneficial aid in tracking blood strain, levels of cholesterol, and commonplace cardiovascular fitness.

Preserving maximum great cardiovascular health diminishes the chance of conditions collectively with coronary heart sickness, stroke, and different cardiovascular illnesses. It includes an entire method that integrates way of life options, everyday bodily interest, and a coronary coronary heart-healthy food regimen. Consistent clinical checkups and consultations with healthcare providers are vital for tracking and keeping cardiovascular health

Cardiovascular workout and its characteristic in muscle building and trendy health

Let's discover how cardiovascular exercise contributes to each muscle constructing and ordinary health.

Cardiovascular Exercise and Muscle Building:

Enhanced Blood Circulation:

Cardio activities, along with going for walks or swimming, decorate blood go with the flow, handing over more oxygen and nutrients to muscle businesses for better recuperation and increase.

Caloric Expenditure:

Cardiovascular physical sports activities burn electricity, assisting fats loss and in a roundabout way supporting muscle definition.

Heart Health Impact:

A sturdy cardiovascular system improves blood pumping in some unspecified time in the future of exercising, reaping blessings general ordinary overall performance, in conjunction with muscle-building sports activities.

Increased Endurance:

Improved cardiovascular fitness boosts endurance at some stage in resistance schooling, facilitating greater reps and units for muscle improvement.

Cardiovascular Exercise and Overall Health:

Heart Health Benefits:

Regular aerobic strengthens the coronary heart, decreasing the risk of cardiovascular troubles like coronary heart attacks and strokes.

Weight Management:

Cardio contributes to calorie burning, helping in weight control for conventional health.

Blood Pressure Regulation:

Cardio bodily games help regulate blood strain, lowering the hazard of excessive blood pressure.

Cholesterol Control:

Cardio promotes a healthy cholesterol stability, with extended HDL and reduced LDL, helping coronary heart fitness.

Mood and Mental Health Improvement:

Cardio sports release endorphins, lowering pressure and improving mood, contributing to higher highbrow fitness.

Respiratory Function Enhancement:

Cardio sporting sports enhance lung potential and breathing characteristic, helping everyday breathing fitness.

Blood Sugar Management:

Cardio aids in blood sugar law, decreasing the threat of kind 2 diabetes and supporting metabolic fitness.

Boosted Energy Levels:

Regular cardiovascular exercise can growth strength stages, enhancing each day functioning.

Balancing Cardio and Muscle Building:

Frequency: Strive for a balance amongst cardio and resistance education, adjusting primarily based on individual dreams and alternatives.

Intensity: Modify depth in your goals, considering excessive-depth c language training (HIIT) for each cardiovascular health and calorie expenditure.

Rest and Recovery: Allow sufficient relaxation amongst aerobic and muscle-building instructions to prevent overtraining.

In summary, cardiovascular exercise plays a important function in supporting muscle constructing, promoting average health, and presenting blessings to the cardiovascular tool. It's important for preserving nicely-being and achieving fitness dreams.

Chapter 14: The Role of Rest and Recovery

Rest and recovery are similar to the unsung heroes in the epic tale of muscle constructing. You see while you hit the health club and supply the ones muscle mass a super exercise, you are inviting them to expand stronger. But here's the seize: the real magic happens even as you're no longer pumping iron.

During rest, your frame goes into repair mode. It's like a production group fixing up the wear and tear and tear out of your severe exercise. Without right rest, it is like interrupting the construction people earlier than they stop the manner. They need their espresso ruin too, ?

Now, on the subject of muscle building in guys, it is vital to permit those muscles get higher. That way getting sufficient sleep, taking days off amongst intense sporting activities, and probably even throwing in some relaxation techniques. It's not approximately being lazy; it's miles about giving your muscle businesses the VIP treatment they deserve.

Imagine your muscle mass as a collection of superheroes. They exit and combat the villains in the gymnasium, however additionally they need their downtime in the thriller lair to recharge and are to be had returned stronger. So, rest isn't handiest a luxury; it is a need in case you need those muscle businesses to reach their whole capability.

In the arena of muscle building, the actual earnings appear on the equal time as you're catching a few Zs or lounging at the couch with a protein shake in hand. So, my friend, include the energy of rest and recuperation— it's far the decision of the sport weapon within the quest for powerful muscle tissues!

Preventing Common Injuries in Men's Muscle Building

The the darkish aspect of muscle building— commonplace injuries. It's like navigating a battlefield, however with dumbbells in preference to swords. Let's shed a few moderate on the ones ability pitfalls:

1.   Strains and Sprains: These are just like the ninja assassins of the muscle international. Strains seem on the same time as a muscle or tendon gets stretched or torn, on the identical time as sprains involve ligaments. So, it is like your muscle groups and connective tissues are doing acrobatics they may be not organized for.

2.   Tendonitis: Think of tendons due to the fact the bridge amongst muscle and bone. When they get indignant or inflamed, it is tendonitis. It's like the bridge toll collector is on strike, inflicting traffic jams and chaos.

3.   Overuse Injuries: Too masses of an terrific problem may be horrible. Overtraining without giving your muscle groups the risk to get better is a one-way price tag to overuse accidents. It's like making your muscle tissues paintings past normal time without any weekends off.

four.   Strained Back: Deadlifts and squats are similar to the rockstars of muscle constructing bodily activities. But if you don't bring with right shape, your decrease once more might probably enjoy find it impossible to resist just went through a mosh pit.

5.   Rotator Cuff Injuries: Shoulder muscle tissue, in particular the rotator cuff, can take a beating in case you're not cautious collectively together with your shoulder carrying activities. It's like having a sensitive flower in your garden—cope with it with care, or it'd wither.

6.   Shin Splints: Not splendid to runners, shin splints can also pay a visit to the ones doing excessive leg bodily video games. It's like your shins are throwing a protest because they're now not getting the attention they deserve.

HOW TO AVOID INJURIES

nine The key to keeping off these accidents is a balanced method. Warm-up well, use right shape, don't overtrain, and throw in a few rest days. It's like developing a castle to defend your gains from the lurking dangers of muscle-building injuries. So, bear in mind, teach smart, and can your earnings be damage-unfastened! How to avoid those injuries Warm up well: Make high quality to spend five-10 minutes warming up in advance than you begin your workout. This have to include mild aerobic, dynamic stretches, and mobility physical games.

10 Start with right shape: Always prioritize well shape over heavy weights. It's higher to boost a lighter weight with right shape than to risk injury with wrong technique.

eleven Progress little by little: Don't rush into lifting heavy weights. Gradually increase the intensity of your workout sporting activities to offer your muscle mass and joints time to evolve.

12 Include relaxation days: Your muscular tissues want time to get better and broaden stronger. Schedule rest days among

immoderate exercising workout routines to prevent overtraining and reduce the danger of injuries.

thirteen Stay hydrated: Dehydration could have an impact in your time-honored overall performance and increase the risk of injuries. Drink sufficient water in the direction of the day, specially throughout bodily games.

14 Listen in your body: Pay interest to any pain or pain. If you experience pain (now not to be pressured with the usual muscle discomfort), it's miles a signal that a few factor is probably incorrect. Rest and are trying to find expert advice if desired.

15 Incorporate variety: Mix up your exercising recurring to keep away from overuse accidents. Include loads of wearing activities that concentrate on specific muscle groups.

Chapter 15: The Importance of Sleep for Men's Health

nine.1 Sleep is a important and essential physiological approach that plays a crucial feature in retaining substantial health and well-being. Here's an proof of sleep and its significance:

1.   Sleep Cycle:

Sleep follows a cyclical pattern, encompassing degrees together with light sleep, deep sleep, and REM (Rapid Eye Movement) sleep. A whole sleep cycle usually lasts 90-110 minutes.

2.   Restoration and Repair:

During sleep, the frame engages in essential restoration and repair processes. This consists of the repair of tissues and muscle organizations, release of increase hormones, and strengthening of the immune device.

three. Memory Consolidation:

Sleep is vital for consolidating reminiscences and facilitating studying. It aids in organizing and storing statistics received at some stage in the day, enhancing cognitive competencies and hassle-solving skills.

four.   Energy Conservation:

Sleep contributes to energy conservation through manner of decreasing the metabolic charge and decreasing body temperature. This conservation is vital for typical physical and intellectual functioning.

five.   Hormone Regulation:

Sleep intricately regulates hormones, in conjunction with the ones governing stress, urge for meals, and growth. Disruptions in sleep can effect hormone stability, essential to severa health troubles.

6.   Mood Regulation:

Adequate sleep is critical for temper regulation, with sleep deprivation associated with irritability, mood swings, and an improved chance of intellectual health conditions which include depression and tension.

7.   Cardiovascular Health:

Chronic sleep deprivation is associated with an progressed danger of cardiovascular illnesses like hypertension and coronary coronary coronary heart assaults. Quality sleep allows coronary coronary heart health and continues wholesome blood stress.

8.   Immune Function:

Sleep is important for a robust immune device. It enhances the producing of cytokines, proteins assisting in immune response, and assists the frame in protecting in competition to infections and ailments.

9.   Weight Management:

Sleep plays a function in regulating urge for food hormones. Lack of sleep is correlated with an prolonged urge for meals, in particular for excessive-calorie and carbohydrate-wealthy elements, contributing to weight benefit.

10.   Physical Performance:

Athletes advantage notably from ok sleep, experiencing advanced response time, superior staying electricity, and usual bodily overall performance.

eleven.   Circadian Rhythm Regulation:

Sleep permits alter circadian rhythms, the frame's internal clock, contributing to higher full-size fitness and functioning.

12.   Brain Health:

Sleep is important for mind health, helping neuroplasticity—the mind's capacity to evolve and studies new facts. It moreover aids in clearing waste products from the brain.

In summary, sleep is a essential element of a wholesome way of lifestyles, promoting bodily, intellectual, and emotional properly-being. Prioritizing and retaining true sleep behavior are crucial for time-venerated fitness and a excessive splendid of lifestyles.

Effects of lack of sleep on men's Cognitive Impairment:

Sleep deprivation can cause impaired cognitive characteristic, affecting memory, interest, preference-making, and giant mental readability.

Mood Changes:

Lack of sleep is associated with temper disturbances, which incorporates increased irritability, temper swings, and a higher susceptibility to pressure. It can contribute to symptoms and signs and symptoms of hysteria and despair.

Impaired Performance:

Sleep deprivation negatively impacts physical and intellectual ordinary overall overall performance, essential to reduced response time, coordination, and ordinary productivity.

Hormonal Imbalance:

Insufficient sleep can disrupt the stableness of hormones, affecting the release of boom hormone, cortisol (pressure hormone), and intercourse hormones. This imbalance can effect libido, fertility, and muscular tissues.

Weight Gain:

Sleep deprivation is related to an advanced urge for meals, specially for excessive-calorie and sugary food. This can make a contribution to weight benefit and weight problems through the years.

Weakened Immune System:

Chronic loss of sleep compromises the immune gadget, making the body extra vulnerable to infections and illnesses.

Cardiovascular Health Risks:

Sleep deprivation is associated with an extended chance of cardiovascular issues, together with excessive blood strain (excessive blood stress), coronary coronary heart ailment, and stroke.

Impaired Glucose Metabolism:

Insufficient sleep can result in insulin resistance and impaired glucose metabolism, contributing to a sophisticated chance of type 2 diabetes.

Increased Inflammation:

Lack of sleep has been associated with stepped forward infection within the frame, it truely is a aspect in severa continual sicknesses.

Reduced Libido and Sexual Function:

Hormonal imbalances due to sleep deprivation can impact libido and sexual feature in every women and men.

Accelerated Aging:

Chronic sleep deprivation is associated with untimely developing older, affecting pores and pores and skin health, cognitive function, and general strength.

Elevated Stress Levels:

Sleep deprivation can cause prolonged strain ranges, exacerbating emotions of tension and tension.

Risk of Accidents:

Fatigue from lack of sleep impairs motor abilties, reaction time, and preference-making, developing the chance of accidents and accidents.

Hallucinations and Delusions:

Extreme sleep deprivation can cause hallucinations, delusions, and disorientation.

It's critical to be aware that person responses to sleep deprivation can range, and acute periods of sleep loss can regularly be recovered with enough rest. However, continual sleep deprivation might also have cumulative and lengthy-time period effects on fitness. Establishing regular and wholesome sleep behavior is vital for everyday nicely-being. If you are commonly experiencing difficulties with sleep, it's far truly useful to talk over with a healthcare professional for guidance. Anything particular you want to speak about similarly?

9.Three

Maintain a Regular Sleep Schedule:

Go to mattress and wake up on the same time each day to regulate your body's internal clock and decorate sleep extremely good continually.

Establish a Relaxing Bedtime ROUTINE

Develop a chilled regular earlier than sleep, incorporating activities like studying, taking a warmth tub, or operating toward rest strategies to sign your frame that it is time to wind down.

Reduce Screen Time Before Bed:

Minimize publicity to digital gadgets, collectively with smartphones and laptop structures, at the least an hour earlier than bedtime to keep away from disruption of melatonin production.

Optimize Your Sleep Environment:

Create a comfortable and tranquil mattress room with minimal mild, noise, and a groovy temperature. Invest in a excellent mattress and pillows for a greater restful sleep.

Manage Light Exposure:

Expose your self to herbal moderate within the route of the day, especially inside the morning, and dim the lights inside the middle of the night to useful resource your body's herbal sleep-wake cycle.

Monitor Your Diet:

Avoid heavy meals, caffeine, and nicotine close to bedtime to save you disturbances in sleep patterns.

Engage in Regular Exercise:

Incorporate normal bodily hobby into your recurring, however complete your exercising some hours in advance than bedtime to sell better sleep with out interfering with midnight rest.

Practice Stress Management:

Employ strain-lowering techniques collectively with meditation, deep breathing, or innovative muscle rest to enhance relaxation in advance than bedtime.

Limit Napping:

If you want to nap, preserve it short and keep away from sound asleep too near bedtime to prevent disruption of midnight sleep.

Control Liquid Intake Before Bed:

Minimize the intake of liquids, mainly caffeinated and alcoholic beverages, in the hours major as a whole lot as bedtime to reduce the probability of interruptions for lavatory visits.

Explore Natural Remedies:

Consider natural remedies like herbal teas (which include chamomile) or aromatherapy (like lavender) to sell a revel in of rest earlier than sleep.

Consult a Health Professional:

If sleep issues persist, searching for steerage from a healthcare professional to select out out and address capability underlying issues, along with sleep issues.

By incorporating those hints into your ordinary constantly, you could create an environment and behavior conducive to stepped forward sleep outstanding. Patience and commitment to the ones modifications are key

Chapter 16: Mental Health and Stress Management

Mental Health:

Awareness and Stigma Reduction:

Recognizing and acknowledging mental fitness is important. Reducing the stigma surrounding intellectual fitness encourages open conversations and searching out help while needed.

Emotional Expression:

Encouraging the expression of emotions allows save you emotional suppression, fostering higher highbrow fitness. Men are regularly socialized to be stoic, but expressing emotions is vital.

Social Connections:

Maintaining sturdy social connections and fostering supportive relationships absolutely affects intellectual fitness. Regular social interactions provide a experience of belonging and resource.

Healthy Lifestyle Choices:

A balanced food plan, normal exercising, and sufficient sleep contribute to intellectual properly-being. Physical health and highbrow health are interconnected.

Seeking Professional Help:

Recognizing the significance of expert highbrow health aid is vital. Therapists, counselors, and psychologists can offer treasured help for intellectual fitness demanding situations.

Mindfulness and Meditation:

Practices like mindfulness and meditation sell highbrow clarity, lessen strain, and beautify ordinary nicely-being.

Stress Management:

Identifying Stressors:

Understanding belongings of stress allows proactive manipulate. Identifying stressors permits increase powerful coping techniques.

Time Management:

Efficient time manage reduces the pressure of closing dates, minimizing strain. Prioritize duties and set practical wants to keep away from feeling overwhelmed.

Physical Activity:

Regular workout is a powerful pressure reducer. Physical interest releases endorphins, the body's herbal temper lifters, and offers an outlet for accumulated anxiety.

Relaxation Techniques:

Incorporate relaxation techniques at the facet of deep breathing, present day muscle relaxation, or guided imagery into your normal to control strain successfully.

Balancing Work and Personal Life:

Establish clean limitations among work and personal existence. Striking a stability guarantees that one aspect does not dominate, major to persistent stress.

Healthy Coping Mechanisms:

Avoid terrible coping mechanisms like excessive alcohol intake or tobacco use. Instead, interact in sports sports that deliver satisfaction and rest.

Setting Realistic Expectations:

Setting viable dreams and expectancies prevents useless stress. Recognize and characteristic a very good time small successes in area of fixating on perfection.

Social Support:

Sharing problems with pals, circle of relatives, or a aid network can provide mindset and emotional guide sooner or later of stressful times.

Mind-Body Connection:

Practices like yoga or tai chi emphasize the mind-body connection, promoting relaxation and reducing stress.

Cognitive Behavioral Techniques:

Cognitive-behavioral treatment (CBT) techniques assist reframe bad concept styles, fostering a more exceptional outlook and decreasing strain.

Prioritizing highbrow health and adopting powerful pressure control techniques make contributions to a more healthy and extra satisfying life. Seeking help even as wanted is a sign of power, no longer vulnerable point. If you or someone you apprehend is suffering with intellectual fitness, expert assistance is available and useful.

Supplements for Men's Muscle Building

While it is critical to attain crucial nutrients from a nicely-rounded diet regime, some men may also moreover consider dietary dietary dietary supplements to resource in muscle constructing. Here are numerous nutritional supplements normally related to muscle improvement:

Protein Supplements:

Whey Protein: Quickly absorbed for placed up-exercise restoration.

Casein Protein: Digested slowly, imparting a sustained launch of amino acids.

Branched-Chain Amino Acids (BCAAs):

Essential amino acids like leucine, isoleucine, and valine resource protein synthesis and muscle restoration.

Creatine:

Creatine monohydrate, a nicely-researched supplement, complements energy, muscle tissues, and gives power throughout extreme workout routines.

Beta-Alanine:

Aids in developing muscle carnosine ranges, buffering acid, and delaying fatigue at some point of excessive-depth exercise.

L-Glutamine:

An amino acid supporting muscle restoration and immune feature, usually used within the route of extreme schooling intervals.

Omega-3 Fatty Acids:

Found in fish oil, omega-3s provide anti inflammatory blessings and manual joint health vital for education.

Vitamin D:

Essential for bone fitness, nutrition D can also play a feature in muscle function and testosterone degrees.

Zinc and Magnesium:

Important minerals worried in severa physiological strategies, including hormone manufacturing and muscle characteristic.

Vitamin C and E:

Antioxidant nutrients which consist of C and E lessen oxidative strain from intense exercise, assisting in recuperation.

Beta-Hydroxy Beta-Methylbutyrate (HMB):

A leucine metabolite, HMB can also help decrease muscle protein breakdown and resource muscle increase.

It's vital to consider that the ones nutritional dietary supplements should complement a balanced eating regimen and proper schooling routine. Individual desires variety, and consulting with a healthcare professional or registered dietitian earlier than which includes dietary dietary supplements is simply beneficial. Additionally, display the superb and dosage of supplements to save you functionality damaging results. A properly-rounded weight-reduction plan with sufficient strength, protein, carbohydrates, and fats stays the cornerstone of effective muscle building.

Common Health Concerns for Men and How to Address Them

Here are some everyday health problems for men and strategies to address them:

Heart Health:

Addressing Concern: Embrace a coronary coronary coronary heart-healthful way of life through preserving a well-balanced eating regimen, collaborating in regular workout, handling stress, and steerage smooth of tobacco use.

Prostate Health:

Addressing Concern: Regularly time table test-u.S.A.With a healthcare provider, mainly as you age. Discuss prostate health screenings and incorporate a diet regime rich in quit quit end result, veggies, and omega-3 fatty acids.

Testicular Health:

Addressing Concern: Conduct normal testicular self-tests for early detection of abnormalities. Seek spark off clinical hobby for any adjustments or problems.

Mental Health:

Addressing Concern: Prioritize intellectual well-being through trying to find manual whilst wanted, fostering sturdy social connections, training pressure control techniques, and thinking about therapy or counseling.

Weight Management:

Addressing Concern: Adopt a balanced food regimen, have interaction in regular physical pastime, and control difficulty sizes. Consult with a healthcare organization for custom designed weight control steering.

Diabetes Prevention:

Addressing Concern: Sustain a healthful weight, participate in ordinary workout, and show blood sugar degrees. Regular test-united statesresource in early detection and manage of diabetes.

Colon Health:

Addressing Concern: Schedule habitual screenings for colorectal most cancers, mainly with a own family data. Maintain a excessive-fiber diet and stay hydrated for advanced colon health.

Bone Health:

Addressing Concern: Consume enough calcium and nutrition D thru diet or supplements. Engage in weight-bearing physical video video games to assist bone health and mitigate the threat of osteoporosis.

Sexual Health:

Addressing Concern: Maintain open verbal exchange with healthcare vendors regarding sexual fitness issues. Seek scientific steering for addressing erectile dysfunction.

Lung Health:

Addressing Concern: Quit smoking if relevant, keep away from exposure to secondhand smoke, and recollect of workplace or environmental factors affecting lung health.

Vision Health:

Addressing Concern: Schedule ordinary eye checks for monitoring and early detection. Safeguard your eyes from UV rays, and uphold a balanced diet regime for everyday eye health.

Skin Health:

Addressing Concern: Shield your pores and skin from solar publicity using sunscreen and shielding apparel. Monitor moles for adjustments and go through everyday skin tests with a dermatologist.

Hypertension (High Blood Pressure):

Addressing Concern: Regularly show display screen blood pressure, undertake a low-sodium weight loss plan, have interaction in everyday exercising, and control pressure to prevent or manage excessive blood pressure.

Consistent check-ups, screenings, and a proactive method to a wholesome way of life drastically make a contribution to preventing and addressing those regularly occurring health concerns for guys. If you have particular inquiries or issues, consulting with a healthcare professional is truly beneficial.